BUTTERWORTH
HEINEMANN'S

Review
Questions
for the NBEO®
EXAMINATION

PART TWO

D1568522

BUTTERWORTH
HEINEMANN'S

Review
Questions
for the NBEO®
EXAMINATION
PART TWO

Edited by

Edward S. Bennett, OD, MSEd

Associate Professor
Director, Student Services
Co-Chief, Contact Lens Service
College of Optometry
University of Missouri–St. Louis
St. Louis, Missouri

Vasudevan Lakshminarayanan, PhD

Associate Professor of Optometry
Associate Professor of Physics and Astronomy
College of Optometry
University of Missouri–St. Louis
St. Louis, Missouri

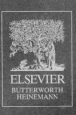
ELSEVIER
BUTTERWORTH
HEINEMANN

BUTTERWORTH
HEINEMANN
ELSEVIER

11830 Westline Industrial Drive
St. Louis, Missouri 63146

Notice

Buterworth Heinemann's Review Questions for the NBEO® Examination: Part Two is a resource for optometric students preparing to take the NBEO® examination, state or local boards, as well as for the optometrist seeking state licensure. The publisher makes no claims regarding the effectiveness or relevance of the content or presentation of this material and makes no guarantee regarding any individual's performance on any of these examinations.

ISBN-13: 978-0-7506-7566-6
ISBN-10: 0-7506-7566-7

Publishing Director: Linda Duncan
Acquisitions Editor: Kathy Falk
Senior Developmental Editor: Christie M. Hart
Publishing Services Manager: Patricia Tannian
Project Manager: Sarah Wunderly
Design Direction: Kathi Gosche

Printed in United States of America

Last digit is the print number: 9   8   7   6   5   4   3   2   1

To our students, past, present, and future
ESB and VL

To my family: my wife, Jean, my children, Matt, Josh, and Emily, my sister, Holly,
and my mother, Mary Edith Snider
ESB

To Nan and the girls, my stellini
VL

Contributors

Greg Black, OD
Assistant Professor of Optometry
Primary Care Service
Eye Institute, Broward Clinic
Nova Southeastern University
Ft. Lauderdale, Florida

Robert Buckingham, OD, PhD
Director of Clinics
Michigan College of Optometry
Ferris State University
Big Rapids, Michigan

Michelle Caputo, OD
Optometric Director
Neuro-ophthalmology Service
Bascom Palmer Eye Institute
Miami, Florida

Elise B. Ciner, OD, FAAO
Associate Clinical Professor
Department of Pediatrics and
    Binocular Vision
Pennsylvania College of Optometry
Elkins Park, Pennsylvania

John G. Classé, OD, JD
School of Optometry
University of Alabama at
    Birmingham
Birmingham, Alabama

John B. Crane, OD
Clinical Assistant Professor
College of Optometry
University of Missouri—St. Louis
St. Louis, Missouri

Dawn DeCarlo, OD, MS
Associate Professor
College of Optometry
Nova Southeastern University
Ft. Lauderdale, Florida

John R. Griffin, MOpt, OD, MSEd
Distinguished Professor Emeritus
Southern California College of
    Optometry
Fullerton, California

Michael P. Keating, PhD
Professor
Michigan College of Optometry
Ferris State University
Big Rapids, Michigan

Kelly A. Malloy, OD, FAAO
Assistant Professor
Pennsylvania College of Optometry
Elkins Park, Pennsylvania
Director
Neuro-Ophthalmic Disease Clinical
    Speciality Service
The Eye Institute of the Pennsylvania
    College of Optometry
Philadelphia, Pennsylvania

James R. Miller, OD
Professor
Michigan College of Optometry
Ferris State University
Big Rapids, Michigan

Bruce Morgan, OD, FAAO
Chief of Cornea and Contact Lens
  Services, Associate Professor
Michigan College of Optometry
Ferris State University
Big Rapids, Michigan

Gale Orlansky, OD
Assistant Professor
Pennsylvania College of Optometry
Elkins Park, Pennsylvania

Jennifer A. Palombi, OD
Adjunct Clinical Faculty
College of Optometry
The Ohio State University
Columbus, Ohio
Clinical Consultant
Eye Clinic
Department of Veterans Affairs
  Medical Center
Dayton, Ohio

Nancy Peterson-Klein, OD
Associate Dean for Academic and
  Student Affairs, Professor of
  Optometry
Michigan College of Optometry
Ferris State University
Big Rapids, Michigan

Lewis Reich, OD, PhD, FAAO
Assistant Dean for Student Affairs
College of Optometry
Nova Southeastern University
Ft. Lauderdale, Florida

Daniel K. Roberts, OD, MS
Professor of Optometry
Illinois Eye Institute
Illinois College of Optometry
Chicago, Illinois

Leo P. Semes, OD, FAAO
Associate Professor
School of Optometry
University of Alabama at
  Birmingham
Birmingham, Alabama

Brad M. Sutton, OD, FAAO
Indiana University School of
  Optometry
Clinic Director
Indianapolis Eye Care Center
Indianapolis, Indiana

Julie Tyler, OD, FAAO
Assistant Professor of Optometry
Chief of Primary Care at Davie
  College of Optometry
Nova Southeastern University
Ft. Lauderdale, Florida

Philip E. Walling, OD, FAAO
Professor
Michigan College of Optometry
Ferris State University
Big Rapids, Michigan

Chris Woodruff, OD, MBA, FAAO
Associate Professor of Optometry
Nova Southeastern University
Ft. Lauderdale, Florida

Albert D. Woods, MS, OD, FAAO
Director of Electrodiagnostic Service
Associate Professor
College of Optometry
Nova Southeastern University
Ft. Lauderdale, Florida

Preface

For the Prospective Test-Taker

This book is intended to be an important resource in your preparation for the National Board of Examiners in Optometry (NBEO®) Part Two examination. This examination is very challenging because of the vast amount of material covering systemic conditions, ocular disease, refractive, oculomotor and sensory integrative conditions, perceptual conditions, public health, and legal and ethical issues that you must master. It is important to emphasize that this text represents only one of many resources a student should use in preparing for this examination. There is no substitute for extensive preparation, which should begin soon after you enter the optometric program. This book should represent a check of your mastery of the various subject areas.

One of the first steps in preparing for the NBEO® examination is to review the NBEO Part Two content outline. Updates are available from the NBEO® website (www.optometry.org). You should carefully review the primary topics and the subtopics listed, as well as the potential number of questions that will be provided in each of these areas. As a student, you should take comprehensive and legible notes in the pertinent optometric courses during your first 3 years in the optometric program. These notes should be well organized and easy to read for future review. It cannot be emphasized enough that there is far too much information to memorize when preparing for this examination; therefore, it is extremely important to learn the material in the classroom to facilitate recall for the NBEO® examination. Material that was never learned or understood is material that will be difficult to learn or memorize at a later date.

The timing of your review for this examination is individual in nature; however, most students cannot begin early enough. The summer after the third year of optometry school should be devoted to organizing notes in the content areas, as well as writing out quiz questions within each subtopic area. A second option would be to organize this material as well as quiz questions (the use of index cards with on-line questions is recommended), although adherence to a strict schedule can be difficult because of the rigors of the clinical curriculum. It is important to use many different resources (e.g., lecture notes, texts, study guides) when preparing for every section of the examination. Using this information to write out examination questions is beneficial because learning is greater if you recite information aloud as opposed to devoting all of your time to reading the pertinent information.

How you prepare is important as well. From our experience and from talking with students, we found that most students benefit from study groups.

A group of two to four students can meet on a weekly basis during the few months immediately before the examination (although they certainly could initiate the process much earlier). A new topic should be scheduled to be reviewed each week with the subsections of that topic divided among the members of the group. Each member could develop a series of questions within his or her topic, and the weekly meeting could be an excellent opportunity to quiz one another on this material.

Develop a study plan for the more intense review scheduled for the final 8 to 10 weeks before the examination. This plan should be a realistic one that allows for the inevitable interruptions (e.g., illness, family obligations, part-time employment) that can occur. Review your progress on compliance with this schedule on a weekly basis; if you are not able to meet the demands of the schedule, determine possible ways that your time could be better devoted to the schedule (i.e., minimize "time-wasters").

Also important is where and when you study. You cannot retain information in front of a television, in a noisy environment, or in an environment in which distractions are inevitable. Studying in a quiet place during the time of day that you are most alert and capable of learning is recommended. As the amount of material to be reviewed during this time is extensive, the schedule should represent a primary focus of every student to increase the likelihood of success. It is often beneficial to study the most difficult material first with the last 3 weeks representing a very intense review of all material.

During the examination itself it is important to think positively. Everyone will be apprehensive. It is vital not to worry about those around you. You should resist all distractions and have confidence in your ability. It is important to keep your focus on the examination itself, not the consequences. From time to time look away, take a deep breath, and relax. The mental strain of such a lengthy examination necessitates this action. Remember to budget your time appropriately. Determine how many questions there are for a designated amount of time and divide by the number of questions (leaving some time for review at the end as well) to determine the correct pace for answering all of the questions.

Read every question and answer option very carefully. This is crucial because most answer choices include what are termed "sophisticated distractors." These are answer options that are similar to the correct answer. Often, a question is answered incorrectly because the test-taker overlooks a word such as "not" in this example: "Which one of the following is NOT representative of this condition?" Another way to avoid the pitfall of the sophisticated distractor is to cover up the answer choices, work out the correct answer, and then see which one of the choices corresponds to the answer you have determined.

Because you can miss a large number of questions and still pass the examination, do not become discouraged if you encounter a series of questions for which you are not sure of the correct response. If you are unsure, make the best educated guess possible, review it at the conclusion of the examination, and only change your response if you are absolutely certain the revised response is more likely to be correct. Another good reason to review all of your answers is the possibility of failing to record an answer or, worse yet, having your answers out of sequence (e.g., your answer to #13 was recorded as #12). Do not spend an inordinate amount of time on any one question. If the question is very challenging, move to the next question and wait until near the end of the examination to answer the most difficult questions.

It is our sincere hope that you will find this text to be one of many useful resources in your preparation for the NBEO® Part Two examination. The CD-ROM will allow you to practice taking mock examinations (make sure to time yourself during the mock examination) and—in addition to the book and frequent quizzing by yourself and others—allow you to approach this challenging examination with confidence.

Acknowledgments

The editors would like to thank Sarah Wunderly, Project Manager at Elsevier, for her assistance in this project.

It is very important to emphasize that this text—as well as the NBEO Part One text—were made possible through the tireless efforts of Christie Hart, Senior Developmental Editor at Elsevier, who originated these projects and solicited several of the contributing authors. The editors, as well as the optometric profession, are grateful to have someone of her vision and dedication.

Contents

Part 2   Ocular Disease and Trauma

Part 3   Refractive, Oculomotor, Sensory, and Integrative Conditions

Systemic Conditions

CHAPTER 1

General Health

Albert D. Woods, Greg Black, Julie Tyler, Michelle Caputo

1. Homocysteine is being used with increasing frequency in health screenings to help evaluate certain health risk factors. All of the following are true about homocysteine EXCEPT:
   a. high levels of homocysteine are associated with atherosclerosis with an increased risk of coronary artery disease
   b. high levels of homocysteine are associated with high levels of B vitamins
   c. high levels of homocysteine can promote blood clot formation in the deep veins of the legs (i.e., deep venous thrombosis)
   d. high levels of homocysteine can occur in patients with renal compromise/failure

2. Which of the following conditions is(are) associated with fatigue?
   a. anemia
   b. hypothyroidism
   c. hyperthyroidism
   d. a and b
   e. a, b, and c

3. All of the following are considered normal developmental milestones EXCEPT:
   a. has vertical eye coordination at ≈1 month
   b. visually recognizes mother at ≈2 months
   c. has limited vocabulary of 4 to 6 words including names at ≈10 months
   d. walks unassisted at ≈12 months

4. In performing basic cardiovascular life support, you should:
   a. check for breathing as the first step
   b. initiate breathing if not present with two quick breaths
   c. check circulation after breathing has been assessed, or after the initial two breaths if no breathing was present
   d. give chest compressions at a ratio of 10 compressions to two breaths

5. Alphagan, which is used in the management of glaucoma, has been associated with which systemic side effect(s)?
    a. bradycardia
    b. hypotension
    c. taste alteration
    d. fatigue
    e. a, b, c, and d

6. Although vitamin supplementation is often used in the area of preventive medicine, which vitamin is NOT recommended as a supplement in patients who are heavy smokers?
    a. vitamin C
    b. beta-carotene
    c. vitamin E
    d. folic acid

7. Which of the following migraine types is most commonly associated with a history of marked vertigo?
    a. cerebral migraine
    b. childhood migraine
    c. ophthalmoplegic migraine
    d. basilar migraine

8. Which of the following statements regarding fever is(are) TRUE?
    a. fever is defined as an elevated body temperature above 38.3° C
    b. causes of fever to be considered in a person who travels internationally include malaria, dengue, typhoid, and rickettsial infections
    c. the most reliable body temperature is an oral temperature
    d. a and b
    e. a, b, and c

9. All of the following are systemic side effects of topical nonsteroidal anti-inflammatory drugs (NSAIDs) such as Voltaren or Acular EXCEPT:
    a. gastrointestinal symptoms
    b. exacerbation of asthma
    c. headaches
    d. facial edema
    e. hypertension

10. You have just attended your first national continuing education conference. In one of the lectures, a new screening test was described that can detect early herpes simplex infections. You rarely see herpes simplex in your patient population. You contact other physicians in your area, and they indicate that herpes simplex is known to be rare in the area in which you practice. How would this affect the positive predictive value of this new test for use in your office?
    a. would increase the predictive value of the test results being correct
    b. would decrease the predictive value of the test results being correct
    c. there would be no effect on the predictive value of the test
    d. predictive values are not used when evaluating laboratory tests

11. Which of the following is the most common cause/form of vertigo?
    a. benign paroxysmal positional vertigo (BPPV)
    b. Meniere's disease
    c. trauma
    d. infection

12. Which medication is the drug of choice today for the treatment of the more common migraine types?
    a. ergotamine
    b. dihydroergotamine
    c. amitriptyline
    d. sumatriptan
    e. verapamil

13. Oral corticosteroid drugs are being prescribed more frequently by doctors of optometry in the primary eye-care setting. All of the following are possible side effects of oral corticosteroids prescribed for short-term use (days to a few weeks) EXCEPT:
    a. weight gain
    b. increased blood glucose
    c. fat deposits on the face and back
    d. increased blood pressure
    e. headache

14. Which of the following statements regarding malaise is(are) TRUE?
    a. it is a generalized feeling of discomfort or lack of well-being
    b. fatigue is often found in association with malaise
    c. it can occur with significant infectious, endocrine, neoplastic, or systemic disorders
    d. onset may be slow or rapid
    e. a, b, c, and d

15. All of the following body habitus changes occur in HIV-positive patients on long-term HAART (highly active antiretroviral therapy) EXCEPT:
    a. fat accumulation in the dorsocervical region (i.e., "buffalo hump")
    b. fat accumulation in the abdominal region
    c. loss of subcutaneous fat in the buttocks and the extremities
    d. hair fragility

16. All of the following are consistent with a diagnosis of migraine headaches EXCEPT:
    a. headache sometimes starts on the opposite side of head
    b. aura lasts ≈20 minutes
    c. aura occurs prior to headache
    d. scintillating scotoma forms just off fixation and does not expand
    e. onset before age 20

Answers

1. b. High levels of homocysteine, a natural compound that is derived from dietary proteins, cause injury and scarring to the lining of the blood vessel walls; this leads to stenosis or sometimes complete closure of the arteries affected. Foods rich in B vitamins, including folic acid, vitamin B_6, and vitamin B_{12}, can REDUCE high homocysteine plasma levels.

2. e. While most associate fatigue with hypothyroidism due to the overall metabolic slowdown, it also occurs with hyperthyroidism, usually being noted at the end of the day. Many diseases can have associated fatigue, including anemia, Addison's disease, respiratory allergies (e.g., hay fever), systemic infections, heart failure, diabetes, chronic liver or kidney failure, autoimmune diseases, sleep disorders, and cancer.

3. c. A limited vocabulary and recognizing some names do not show up until around 14 months, so at 10 months this would be advanced development. Other vocabulary milestones are using two-word sentences at 24 months and using complete simple sentences at 36 months.

4. c. In the ABCDs of basic cardiovascular life support, checking the *A*irway is the first step, followed by assessing *B*reathing; if not present, then two slow breaths are given. The next step is to assess *C*irculation and, if absent, then compressions are given at a ratio of 15 compressions to 2 breaths. If an automated external defibrillator is available, then once set up and attached, compressions are stopped and *D*efibrillation is attempted up to 3 times.

5. e. All of the systemic side effects listed for Alphagan have been reported since it became available for clinical use. Because bradycardia, hypotension, hypothermia, hypotonia, and apnea have all been reported in infants on Alphagan, it is not recommended for pediatric patients.

6. b. The U.S. Preventive Services Task Force recommends against the use of beta-carotene supplements in heavy smokers based on the results of two large clinical trials (Beta-Carotene Prevention Study and Beta-Carotene and Retinol Efficacy Trial) where beta-carotene supplementation was associated with a higher incidence of lung cancer and higher mortality rate in smokers.

7. d. Vertigo is the most common symptom associated with a basilar migraine, a migraine variant that is classified as a complicated migraine. The aura phase, including the vertigo, is due to transient brainstem and cerebellar ischemia, which is sometimes mistaken for a transient ischemic attack involving the vertebrobasilar circulation.

8. d. The average body temperature is 36.7° C (range, 36.0° to 37.4° C), with temperatures above 38.3° C being defined as fever. While there are many causes of fever in travelers returning to the United States, particularly in those who have visited undeveloped countries, four of the most common causes of fever include malaria, dengue, typhoid, and rickettsial infections. The most accurate body temperature that is used clinically is the rectal temperature.

9. e. Hypertension is associated with ocular decongestants such as Naphazoline, not with topical nonsteroidal anti-inflammatory drugs (NSAIDs). Because of the potential increase in bleeding time, care is used in patients already taking either oral NSAIDs or steroids. These medications should also be used with care, or not used at all, in patients who are sensitive to aspirin or who have asthma and nasal polyps.

10. b. The positive predictive value is the probability that the test is correct, based on the prevalence of a disease. Thus, in the case of this new screening test, a lower prevalence would decrease the predictive value of the test results being correct, wasting time and money of both the physician and the patient.

11. a. Benign paroxysmal positional vertigo (BPPV) is the most common cause of vertigo and is caused by crystals of debris accumulating in the semicircular canals of the inner ear. The vertigo sensation often starts suddenly, is triggered by head movement, and can show fatigability where after several repetitions of the same head movement the vertigo may no longer occur, until repeated later in the day.

12. d. While all the medications listed can be used in the treatment of migraines, sumatriptan (Imitrex) is currently the drug of choice for relieving the pain and symptoms during a migraine attack. It is available in a tablet, nasal spray, or injection form. Because it constricts blood vessels, it is not used for basilar or hemiplegic migraines or in patients with a history of certain heart conditions, stroke or transient ischemic attacks, or circulatory problems.

13.   c.   While there can be a weight gain with short-term use of oral corticosteroids, actual deposits of fat on the face and back (e.g., buffalo hump) are long-term side effects that take months to years to occur and usually do not go away completely after the medication is stopped.

14.   e.   All of the items listed are consistent with malaise, a nonspecific symptom that can occur with almost any significant systemic disease.

15.   d.   Hair fragility is associated with the wasting syndrome frequently observed in HIV-positive patients before the availability of HAART. The other findings listed are consistent with the lipohypertrophy and lipoatrophy that occurs with long-term HAART. In addition to the body habitus (i.e., body physique or build) changes, there are associated metabolic changes including hypercholesterolemia, hypertriglyceridemia, and hyperglycemia.

16.   d.   The scintillating scotoma seen with a migraine attack starts at fixation and then slowly expands toward the peripheral visual field while fading over 10 to 20 minutes. The term "scintillating scotoma" describes the characteristic flickering of the luminous migraine spectra and is due to a spreading depression wave where neuronal depolarization is followed by neuronal suppression as the wave spreads slowly across the surface of the brain, starting at the occipital cortex.

CHAPTER 2

Neurologic System

Albert D. Woods, Greg Black, Julie Tyler,
Michelle Caputo

CONTENT AREAS

- Epidemiology
- Nonocular neurologic conditions: signs and symptoms
- Laboratory and imaging tests
- Diagnoses and treatment approaches

1. A patient experiences sensory and motor neglect on the left side of the body with problems buttoning the shirt pocket on that same side. An asymmetric optokinetic nystagmus with a reduced response is noted when the stimulus is moved toward the patient's right side. The lesion is located in the:
   a. right parietal lobe
   b. left parietal lobe
   c. right temporal lobe
   d. left temporal lobe

2. A patient presents with a sudden "electric" sensation radiating down the spine when flexing the neck downward toward the chest. The name of this clinical finding is:
   a. Cogan's sign
   b. Uhtoff's phenomenon
   c. Babinski sign
   d. Lhermitte's sign

3. Which of the following statements is FALSE?
   a. interferon B-1a (Avonex) showed no significant effect in delaying the onset of clinically definitive multiple sclerosis (CDMS) in patients who presented with a clinically isolated syndrome typically associated with MS (i.e., optic neuritis)
   b. intravenous methylprednisolone sodium succinate, followed by an oral taper of prednisone, should be given to patients with acute demyelinating optic neuritis with white matter lesions
   c. recombinant interferon B-1a (Rebif) has been found to delay or decrease the incidence of CDMS in patients presenting with their first demyelinating event
   d. a, b, and c are false

4. Which of the following is TRUE about myasthenia gravis (MG)?
    a. blocking antiacetylcholine (ACh) antibodies, binding anti-ACh antibodies, and anti-MuSK (muscle specific kinase) are all diagnostic tests
    b. Mestinon, prednisone, and Cellcept have been used to treat MG
    c. patients with myasthenia gravis should obtain a chest CT scan
    d. the best test to confirm the diagnosis of MG is the Tensilon test
    e. a, b, c, and d are true

5. What test(s) should be initiated with an 86-year-old white woman who presents with severe headaches, weight loss, and jaw claudication?
    a. C-reactive protein (CRP)
    b. erythrocyte sedimentation rate (ESR)
    c. antiphospholipid antibodies
    d. both a and b

6. The degenerative cellular pathology involved in Parkinson's disease is predominantly located in what structure?
    a. substantia nigra
    b. thalamus
    c. cerebellum
    d. pineal gland

7. What is the most potent predictor of clinically definitive multiple sclerosis (CDMS)?
    a. visual acuity
    b. absence of pain
    c. MRI findings
    d. optic disc edema

8. All of the following are true about the Babinski toe sign EXCEPT:
    a. represents an upper motor neuron lesion
    b. represents a pyramidal tract dysfunction
    c. extensor plantar response in which there is dorsiflexion and outward fanning of the big and then the smaller toes
    d. downward flexion of the big toe and then the smaller toes

Answers

1. a. Right-sided parietal lobe lesions usually cause contralateral sensory and motor neglect. The parietal lobe also controls smooth pursuit movements toward the ipsilateral side. Therefore, rotation of the stimulus toward the side of the lesion will demonstrate reduced responses. It is important to note that parietal lobe lesions may or may not have intact visual fields when each hemisphere is tested separately using automated perimetry. However, when a stimulus is presented simultaneously in both hemifields, the patient may only respond to the stimuli in the hemifield ipsilateral to the lesion and show neglect to the contralateral field.

2. d. Lhermitte's sign occurs with flexing of the neck, which produces electric shock–like sensations that extend down the spine and out onto the limbs. This sign occurs in patients who have multiple sclerosis (MS), cervical cord tumors, radiation myelopathy, neck injuries, vitamin B_{12} deficiency, and degenerative changes occurring within the spinal cord.

3. a. The Controlled High Risk Avonex® Multiple Sclerosis Study (CHAMPS) was designed to determine if the treatment with Avonex would benefit patients who had brain signal abnormalities and experienced a first acute demyelinating event involving the optic nerve, brainstem, or spinal cord. The study outcome demonstrated that patients treated with intravenous steroids and once-weekly intramuscular injection of Avonex had a 44% reduction in the 3-year cumulative probability of developing CDMS.

4. e. Traditional acetylcholine (ACh) receptor antibody testing is negative in about 15% of all patients with MG and about 50% of all patients with the pure ocular form of MG. Additional testing in these cases can include binding and blocking ACh receptor antibodies or anti-MuSK antibodies. Tensilon, which blocks the action of acetylcholinesterase, allows more ACh at the neuromuscular junction, causing the ocular or systemic symptoms to improve. Although Mestinon and prednisone are mainstays in the treatment of MG, Cellcept, an immunosuppressive developed to reduce organ rejection, is being used increasingly for severe cases of MG. A chest CT scan should be ordered to rule out a thymoma in MG patients.

5.   d.   The presumed diagnosis of this patient is giant cell arteritis (GCA). GCA can present with multiple symptoms that can include weight loss, jaw claudication, fevers, anemia, myalgias, temporal headaches, and scalp tenderness. The CRP and ESR are the two most important blood tests available in determining GCA. When the CRP and ESR are used together, the specificity for diagnosing GCA approaches 97%; however, the definitive final diagnosis rests on a temporal artery biopsy.

6.   a.   Parkinson's disease results from the degeneration of the dopamine-producing nerve cells in the substantia nigra and the locus ceruleus that send projections to the striatum (putamen). The loss of these cells results in a decreased concentration of endogenous striatal dopamine, which leads to the classic hypokinetic symptoms of Parkinson's. Symptoms typically begin to occur when the dopamine levels fall below 80%.

7.   c.   The 10-year follow-up of the Optic Neuritis Treatment Trial (ONTT) determined that the development of CDMS was significantly associated with one or more white matter lesions on MRI. The 10-year risk of MS was 56% in patients with one or more lesions observed on MRI and 22% in patients who presented with the absence of lesions.

8.   d.   Babinski toe sign is the dorsiflexion (i.e., upward) and/or extension of the big toe, not downward flexion. In many cases there also is fanning of the small toes and, to a lesser degree, dorsiflexion of the ankle and flexion of the hip. Testing involves stroking the sole of the foot with an applicator, starting with the plantar area through the transverse arch to the metatarsophalangeal joint. The Babinski toe sign is associated with upper motor neuron lesions and pyramidal tract lesions.

CHAPTER 3

Musculoskeletal System

*Albert D. Woods, Greg Black, Julie Tyler,
Michelle Caputo*

CONTENT AREAS

- Epidemiology
- Arthritic syndromes: signs and symptoms
- Laboratory and imaging tests
- Diagnoses and treatment approaches

1. All of the following clinical findings are consistent with a diagnosis of ankylosing spondylitis EXCEPT:
   a. anterior nongranulomatous uveitis
   b. negative HLA-B27
   c. lower back pain
   d. sacroiliitis that can lead to kyphosis
   e. posterior synechiae

2. Which onset of juvenile rheumatoid arthritis (JRA) is most likely to have associated ocular findings?
   a. systemic onset
   b. pauciarticular onset
   c. polyarticular onset
   d. there is no association between the type of JRA onset and frequency of ocular findings

3. All of the following are medical treatments that are used in the treatment of systemic lupus erythematosus EXCEPT:
   a. D-penicillamine
   b. hydroxychloroquine
   c. prednisone
   d. cyclophosphamide

4. The CREST syndrome is associated with which disease?
   a. Wegener's granulomatosis
   b. systemic lupus erythematosus
   c. adult rheumatoid arthritis
   d. scleroderma
   e. relapsing polychondritis

5. All of the following findings are consistent with a diagnosis of adult rheumatoid arthritis EXCEPT:
    a. bilateral swollen tender joints
    b. nodules at pressure points
    c. development of osteophytes
    d. elevated gamma globulins (mostly IgM and IgG)

Answers

1. b. Ankylosing spondylitis has the strongest association with HLA B-27, with up to 90% of patients being positive. Other diseases that have a high association with HLA B-27 and can have ocular findings include Reiter's syndrome, inflammatory bowel disease, and psoriatic arthritis.

2. b. Pauciarticular onset, where four or fewer joints are involved, has the greatest association with the anterior uveitis of juvenile rheumatoid arthritis. Both polyarticular onset, in which five or more joints are involved, and systemic onset (i.e., Still's disease), which presents with fever, rash, and lymphadenopathy, have less frequent involvement of the uveitis.

3. a. D-Penicillamine is a degradation product from penicillin that is typically used in the treatment of severe rheumatoid arthritis, Wilson's disease, heavy metal poisoning, and chronic active hepatitis. D-Penicillamine is known to be the cause of drug-induced systemic lupus erythematosus in patients receiving it over a prolonged course of time.

4. d. The CREST syndrome occurs in a subset of patients who present with scleroderma. CREST is an acronym for a series of clinical findings that includes calcinosis, Raynaud's phenomenon, esophageal dysmotility, sclerodactyly, and telangiectasia.

5. c. Osteophytes are abnormal bone growth at joint margins due to loss of joint cartilage from the mechanical wearing down of the joints and are seen in the x-rays of patients with osteoarthritis. They do not occur in rheumatoid arthritis, where joint damage is from inflammation and enzymes found in the joint fluid.

CHAPTER 4

Skin and Hair

Albert D. Woods, Greg Black, Julie Tyler, Michelle Caputo

CONTENT AREAS

- Epidemiology
- Skin manifestation of systemic disorders
- Skin lesions in the phakomatoses
- Common dermatoses
- Skin lesions: benign, premalignant, and malignant
- Medical laboratory tests
- Diagnoses and treatment approaches

1. What systemic condition commonly manifests small, yellowish bumps in rows or a lacy pattern, often on the lateral part of the neck?
   a. systemic lupus erythematosus
   b. pseudoxanthoma elasticum (PXE)
   c. oculocutaneous albinism
   d. syphilis

2. Which of the phakomatoses is associated with a proliferation of neural crest cells and presents with café-au-lait spots, Lisch nodules, and bump-like tumors that grow under the skin?
   a. neurofibromatosis (von Recklinghausen's disease)
   b. Sturge-Weber syndrome
   c. tuberous sclerosis (Bourneville's disease)
   d. ataxia telangiectasia (Louis-Barr syndrome)

3. _____ is an upper respiratory and ocular allergic reaction to airborne substances such as pollen.
   a. atopic dermatitis
   b. allergic contact dermatitis
   c. urticaria
   d. seasonal allergic rhinitis

4. A(n) _____ begins as a round, flesh- or red-colored papule that rapidly progresses to a dome-shaped nodule with a smooth, shiny surface and a central ulceration. It is characterized by rapid growth over a few weeks to months with spontaneous resolution over 4 to 6 months in most cases.
   a. keratoacanthoma
   b. actinic keratosis
   c. malignant melanoma
   d. Kaposi's sarcoma

5. What is the most common sun-related precancerous/cancerous skin lesion?
   a. actinic keratosis
   b. basal cell carcinoma
   c. squamous cell carcinoma
   d. pyogenic granuloma

Answers

1. b. The skin lesions of PXE are characteristic, consisting of small, yellowish bumps in rows or a lacy pattern, which may join to make large patches and are usually noted on the lateral aspect of the neck. The discoid form of lupus erythematosus presents with a red, raised rash primary on the face and scalp. There is also a subacute cutaneous lupus erythematosus where similar lesions appear primarily on the parts of the body exposed to the sun. Red papular lesions may appear with secondary syphilis typically on the palms, soles, trunk, face, and scalp. When oculocutaneous albinism is in its most severe form, the skin and hair remain white throughout life; a less severe form allows the skin and hair to turn slightly darker with age.

2. a. Neurofibromatosis is often diagnosed on the basis of café-au-lait spots, which are irregularly shaped, evenly pigmented, brown macules. Lisch nodules are dome-shaped hamartomas found on the iris surface. Neurofibromas are the most common benign tumor in neurofibromatosis and may be cutaneous, subcutaneous, or plexiform. The cutaneous and subcutaneous lesions are circumscribed nodules that can be soft or firm to touch. Plexiform neurofibromas are noncircumscribed, thick and irregular and are specific to type 1 neurofibromatosis. Sturge-Weber syndrome presents with nevus flammeus (port-wine stain) and cavernous hemangiomas. Tuberous sclerosis has associated adenoma sebaceum (skin angiofibromas) and retinal astrocytic hamartomas. Ataxia telangiectasia can present with telangiectasia of the eyelids, ear, and conjunctiva, along with progressive neurologic impairment and cerebellar ataxia.

3. d. Seasonal allergic rhinitis (i.e., hay fever) is typically caused by an allergy to the pollen of trees, grasses, weeds, or mold spores. It may occur in the spring, summer, or fall and can run a chronic course until the first frost. It presents with sneezing, itching and watery eyes, and a runny nose and is known to trigger asthma. Atopic dermatitis is a chronic skin disease characterized by itchy, inflamed skin with exacerbations and remissions. Poison ivy is a common cause of allergic contact dermatitis, which in the acute stage manifests as redness, bumps, and blisters followed by thickening and scaling. Urticaria is itchy, edematous wheals or red papules that is transient in nature with an intense pruritus.

4. a. Keratoacanthoma is a common low-grade skin cancer that originates in the pilosebaceous glands and pathologically resembles squamous cell carcinoma. It is characterized by rapid growth over weeks to months, followed by spontaneous resolution over 4 to 6 months. Rarely, it can progress to an invasive or metastatic form; because of this, surgical excision is usually advocated. Actinic keratosis usually presents as multiple discrete, flat, or slightly elevated lesions with an erythematous base covered by scales. Malignant melanomas usually present as a flat or slightly elevated brown lesion with irregular pigmentation and borders. Karposi's sarcoma is a tumor that appears reddish or purple on white skin and bluish, brownish or black on dark skin, and is now most commonly observed in association with HIV/AIDS patients.

5. a. Actinic keratosis (or solar keratosis) lesions are precancerous growths that are usually caused by sun exposure and appear as scaly or crusty bumps. They are very common, with approximately 60% of individuals 40 years and older predisposed to have at least one actinic keratosis lesion. Basal cell carcinomas are the most common form of skin cancer and account for 90% of lid cancers. Squamous cell carcinomas are the second most common skin cancer after basal cell carcinoma, and while they usually remain confined to the epidermis, they can extend into the underlying tissues and occasionally metastasize to other organ systems. Pyogenic granulomas are relatively common, benign vascular lesions of the skin and mucosa and usually occur after a minor injury or surgery.

CHAPTER 5

Head and Neck

*Albert D. Woods, Greg Black, Julie Tyler,
Michelle Caputo*

1. A 45-year-old woman presents with pain radiating to the left side of her neck up to her jaw area, along with ptosis and complaints of dysgeusia. On examination, you observe Horner's syndrome on the ipsilateral side of the pain. The diagnosis is which of the following?
   a. temporal arteritis
   b. carotid dissection
   c. migraine
   d. temporomandibular joint disease

2. A patient presents with an asymptomatic carotid occlusion of 65%. What is the proper management for this patient?
   a. carotid endarterectomy
   b. medical
   c. a and b
   d. none of the above

3. Which of the following is the most common cause of a hemifacial spasm?
   a. aneurysms
   b. cerebellopontine angle tumors (CPA)
   c. intraparenchymal brainstem lesions
   d. dolichoectatic vessels compressing on the facial nerve

4. All of the following are true of the trigeminal nerve (CN V) EXCEPT:
   a. it has three major divisions: ophthalmic, maxillary, and mandibular
   b. a cerebellopontine angle tumor can cause paralysis and atrophy of the muscles of mastication leading to loss of strength of bite
   c. the mandibular division of CN V courses through the cavernous sinus
   d. the trigeminal nerve has both a motor and a sensory division

5. An upper motor neuron lesion of the facial nerve (CN VII) on the right side will cause which of the following?
    a. complete facial paralysis of the ipsilateral side of the lesion
    b. complete facial paralysis of the contralateral side of the lesion
    c. paralysis involving the lower half of the face on the contralateral side of the lesion
    d. paralysis on the upper half of the face on the ipsilateral side of the lesion

6. A lower motor neuron lesion of the hypoglossal nerve (CN XII) will cause which of the following?
    a. fasciculation with atrophic changes of the tongue muscle on the ipsilateral side of the lesion; tongue deviates contralateral to the side of the lesion
    b. flaccid paralysis without atrophic changes of the tongue muscles on the contralateral side; tongue deviates to ipsilateral side of lesion
    c. loss of taste of the anterior third of the tongue
    d. loss of taste of the posterior two thirds of tongue

7. Hoarseness and difficulty swallowing are caused by which of the following?
    a. loss of intrinsic muscles of the larynx and loss of the levator palate muscle
    b. endarterectomy, which can cause paralysis of the vocal cord
    c. compromise to the vagus nerve (CN X)
    d. a, b, and c

8. All are true about sensory nerve innervation to the tongue EXCEPT:
    a. general sensory (i.e., pain and temperature) of the anterior two thirds of tongue is innervated by CN V
    b. general sensory to the posterior third of tongue is innervated by the CN IX (glossopharyngeal nerve)
    c. special sensory such as taste of the anterior two thirds of tongue is supplied by CN VII
    d. special sensory of the posterior third of the tongue is supplied by CN XII

Answers

1. b. Carotid dissections may be caused by neck manipulation, trauma following neck or head injury, or spontaneously in cases of fibromuscular dysplasia. Symptoms include pain, which radiates from the neck to the mandibular area or within the orbit. Dysgeusia, which is a metallic taste, occurs if the glossopharyngeal nerve is involved. Diagnosis is made by neuroimaging, either an MRA (magnetic resonance imaging-angiography) or cerebral angiography.

2. c. Surgical management of an asymptomatic carotid occlusion remains controversial. In 1995, the Asymptomatic Carotid Atherosclerosis Study observed that an endarterectomy in patients with asymptomatic carotid occlusions greater than 60% could reduce the incidence of an ipsilateral stroke, although the advantage was small. The American Heart Association recommends consideration of carotid endarterectomy for asymptomatic stenosis of 60% to 99%, in patients with 5-year life expectancy greater than 5%. Medical treatment is also an option, which could include aspirin and/or Plavix or other blood thinners.

3. d. Although all the choices can cause a hemifacial spasm, vascular compression is the main cause in up to 99% of cases. The most common vessels involved are the posterior inferior cerebellar artery, the vertebral artery, and the anterior inferior cerebellar artery. However, because of the potential of an underlying neoplasm or other treatable cause, all patients with hemifacial spasms should undergo neuroimaging studies.

4. c. Within the middle cranial fossa, the trigeminal ganglion divides into three major branches: the ophthalmic (V1), maxillary (V2), and mandibular (V3). Branch V1, and less frequently branch V2, traverses through the cavernous sinus; the mandibular division does not course through the cavernous sinus. The mandibular branch is also different in that it is the only one that has both a sensory and motor division; the other two branches are only sensory.

5. c. Lesions of the upper motor neuron (i.e., brain cortex) cause a paralysis of the contralateral lower face; in this case, the left side. The upper part of the face is spared because it receives innervation from both upper motor neurons; thus, with damage to one side, there is still innervation from the noninvolved side. Stroke is the most common cause of an upper motor neuron lesion involving CN VII.

6. b. The genioglossus muscle of the tongue is the muscle that allows the tongue to project out in a straight-like fashion. The tongue will deviate toward the side of the inactive muscle if one part of the genioglossus muscle is inactive or paralyzed. In a lower motor neuron lesion, the tongue will become flaccid or paralyzed with the tongue deviating ipsilateral to the side of the lesion.

7. d. A lesion of the vagus nerve (CN X) can cause hoarseness, which is due to a unilateral loss of innervation to the intrinsic muscles of the larynx. Causes of unilateral lesions include neoplasms, trauma, or surgical procedures involving the neck such as an endarterectomy. Unilateral loss of the levator palate muscle can be observed by examining the inside of the mouth, noting that the arch of the soft palate will droop on the ipsilateral side of the lesion, causing the uvea to deviate toward the contralateral side.

8. d. Both general sensation and special sensory for the posterior third of the tongue are supplied by CN IX. The hypoglossal nerve (CN XII) supplies motor innervation to the tongue.

CHAPTER 6

Hematopoietic System

*Albert D. Woods, Greg Black, Julie Tyler,
Michelle Caputo*

CONTENT AREAS

- Epidemiology
- Common blood disorders: signs and symptoms
- Laboratory and imaging tests
- Diagnoses and treatment approaches

1. Which of the following statements is INCORRECT regarding total iron binding capacity (TIBC) testing with iron deficiency anemia?
   a. it measures transferrin
   b. it is elevated with iron deficiency
   c. it is depressed with iron deficiency
   d. iron is normally bound to transferrin in blood

2. Patients with Waldenström macroglobulinemia primarily show excessive production of which immunoglobulin?
   a. IgD
   b. IgE
   c. IgG
   d. IgM

3. Which of the following is INCORRECT regarding leukemia?
   a. the hallmark finding of chronic lymphocytic leukemia (CLL) is lymphocytosis of small B-lymphocytes
   b. optic disc edema in leukemia may indicate need for optic nerve irradiation
   c. acute myelocytic leukemia (AML) is the most common form in children
   d. chronic forms of leukemia generally have a poorer prognosis

4. Which test is recommended to follow patients on coumarin therapy because its values are standardized by a reference preparation?
   a. prothrombin time (PT)
   b. partial thromboplastin time (PTT)
   c. international normalized ratio (INR)
   d. free thyroxin index (FTI)

5. General conditions that can cause an INCREASE in RBC count include:
   a. living at a high altitude
   b. certain diseases of the lungs
   c. polycythemia vera
   d. a, b, and c

6. Which of the following combinations of laboratory test results would be most likely to produce an anemic retinopathy in a patient?
   (Hct = hematocrit, PLT = platelets, RBC = red blood cell count)
   a. Hct 35 L (Ref. range: 40% to 54%), PLT 150K (Ref. range: 100 to 400K/µL)
   b. RBC 4 L (Ref. range: 4.5 to 6 mil/µL), PLT 120K (Ref. range: 100 to 400K/µL)
   c. Hct 30 L (Ref. range: 40% to 54%), PLT 110K (Ref. range: 100 to 400K/µL)
   d. RBC 4 L (Ref. range: 4.5 to 6.0 mil/µL), PLT 90K L (Ref. range: 100 to 400K/µL)

7. All of the following statements about hemophilia are correct EXCEPT:
   a. hemophiliacs are deficient in either factor VIII or IX
   b. hemophilia is transmitted as an X-linked recessive trait
   c. ocular manifestations are primarily limited to the anterior segment
   d. classic clinical presentation is pain and swelling in weight-bearing joints due to hemathrosis

8. Which of following statements about Hodgkin's lymphoma is CORRECT?
   a. B-lymphocytes are characterized by the Reed-Sternberg cell
   b. average age of diagnosis is around 67 years
   c. it is likely to appear in the nodes of the abdomen
   d. it accounts for about 85% of all lymphomas

Answers

1. c. TIBC is usually elevated, not depressed, in patients with iron deficiency. With less iron in the blood, there is more free transferring, thus more iron binding sites are available. The elevation of the TIBC is in contrast to two additional tests that are typically run with iron deficiency patients. Both serum ferritin (the major storage form of iron) and serum iron are low in patients with iron deficiency.

2. d. Waldenström macroglobulinemia is characterized by excessive production of monoclonal IgM. It is the overproduction of this large immunoglobulin that increases the blood viscosity and leads to the hyperviscosity changes seen in the retina.

3. c. Acute lymphocytic leukemia (ALL) is the most common form in children, not AML. Although AML can occur in children, it usually occurs in older adults, and with over 10,000 new cases presenting annually, AML is the most common type of acute leukemia in adults. Chronic forms of leukemia generally have a poorer prognosis because symptoms do not present until the disease has reached advanced stages, and many times it is an abnormal laboratory finding, not symptoms, that leads to the diagnostic work-up. With the acute forms, the clinical diagnosis and treatment occur sooner, before the disease advances, because the patients often present complaining about symptoms.

4. c. The INR was developed to reduce the variability in results that occurs when PT is used to monitor Coumadin therapy. The INR standardizes the methods for comparison among different laboratories by running the patient's blood test against a known standard. Typically an INR of 2.5 to 3 indicates the appropriate dosage of Coumadin. Most clinical laboratories still report the PT result along with the INR value, but it is the INR that is being followed clinically.

5. d. All are true. When living at a higher altitude, the body compensates for lower oxygen levels by increasing the number of red blood cells available to carry oxygen picked up at the lungs. Diseases of the lungs that cause hypoxia, such as COPD, will cause the body to compensate by producing more red blood cells. Polycythemia vera is a myeloproliferative disorder of the bone marrow that is characterized by increased red blood cell mass.

6. d. RBC 4 L and PLT 90K L is the only combination given where there is both anemia (as noted by the low RBC level) and thrombocytopenia (noted by the low PLT level). In patients who are both anemic and thrombocytopenic, the likelihood of an anemic retinopathy being present is much higher than if the patient is only anemic or only thrombocytopenic.

7. c. Ocular manifestations of hemophilia are primary neurologic in nature, including papilledema and retrobulbar hemorrhaging or hematoma formation, which can lead to central retinal artery occlusions. While the anterior segment can be involved, such as with a subconjunctival hemorrhage or hyphema, this is a less frequent finding.

8. a. B-lymphocytes are characterized by Reed-Sternberg cells, which are thought to be the neoplastic component in Hodgkin's disease. The other findings listed are more consistent with non-Hodgkin's lymphoma. Hodgkin's lymphoma, in contrast, has an earlier onset with one peak at about 28 years and a smaller secondary peak in patients over the age of 55 years, and it is much less common than non-Hodgkin's lymphoma, accounting for only 15% of all lymphomas.

CHAPTER 7

Immunologic System

Albert D. Woods, Greg Black, Julie Tyler, Michelle Caputo

1. Which of the following AIDS-related opportunistic infections is more marked in the periphery and can rapidly cause full-thickness retinal necrosis leading to retinal detachments as the primary cause of vision loss?
   a. acute retinal necrosis (ARN)
   b. cytomegalovirus retinitis (CMV)
   c. progressive outer retinal necrosis (PORN)
   d. *Candida* retinitis

2. You are seeing a patient who was recently diagnosed with sarcoid after having a chest radiograph performed. A call to the patient's primary care physician indicated that the chest radiograph had shown isolated hilar adenopathy; what pulmonary stage of sarcoid is this?
   a. Stage 0
   b. Stage 1
   c. Stage 2
   d. Stage 3
   e. Stage 4

3. Which of the following findings is consistent with a cytomegalovirus infection?
   a. possible GI system involvement
   b. uveitis
   c. whitish intraretinal lesions with areas of hemorrhaging along the vascular arcades
   d. a, b, and c are possible

4. Which of the following is the most common ocular finding in patients with sarcoid?
   a. candlewax drippings
   b. Koeppe's nodules
   c. lacrimal gland adenitis
   d. anterior uveitis
   e. glaucoma

5. Which of the following drugs, used in the treatment of cytomegalovirus retinitis, carries the highest risk of causing an iritis and/or hypotony?
   a. famciclovir
   b. cidofovir
   c. ganciclovir
   d. foscarnet

6. You are seeing a patient in whom you strongly suspect sarcoidosis. Your initial laboratory evaluation should include all of the following EXCEPT:
   a. chest radiograph
   b. PPD (purified protein derivative)
   c. ACE (angiotensin-converting enzyme)
   d. ANA (antinuclear antibodies)

7. In immediate hypersensitivity allergies, such as allergic rhinoconjunctivitis, which statement is correct about the antibodies that the antigen binds to, which then initiates the immediate response?
   a. found on the surfaces of memory B cells
   b. of the IgM immunoglobulin family
   c. IgG immunoglobulins circulating in the blood
   d. already bound to receptors on mast cells and basophil cells

8. Which of the following laboratory tests would be best to determine the amount of HIV present in the blood of a person?
   a. enzyme-linked immunosorbent assay (ELISA)
   b. Western blot
   c. viral load
   d. P24 antigen

9. A positive tuberculin skin test, with a 15-mm-diameter area of induration on the forearm, appears 72 hours following injection of the PPD. This finding is due to which of the following types of hypersensitivity reaction?
   a. type I hypersensitivity
   b. type II hypersensitivity
   c. type III hypersensitivity
   d. type IV hypersensitivity

10. D4 cell counts in someone with a healthy immune system typically range from:
    a. 10 to 50
    b. 100 to 200
    c. 250 to 350
    d. 500 to 1500

Answers

1. a. The inflammation associated with ARN causes a full-thickness retinal necrosis that leads to a retinal detachment in up to 70% of cases. The two major viruses that cause ARN are herpes zoster and herpes simplex. On a rare occasion, CMV can also be the underlying cause of ARN. While ARN can occur as an opportunistic infection in AIDS patients, this disease is more frequently seen in the nonimmunocompromised patient population. Laser treatment is often performed along the border of the involved retina and noninvolved retina prophylactically to prevent any retinal detachment progression toward the posterior pole.

2. b. Stage 1. There are five stages to the grading system of pulmonary sarcoid. At Stage 0, there are no abnormalities noted on the x-rays. Stage 1 shows only hilar adenopathy with patients typically still asymptomatic at this stage. At Stage 2, the patient usually becomes symptomatic and shows lesions within the lungs along with the hilar adenopathy. By Stage 3, the hilar adenopathy has resolved, but the lung is showing increased lesions on radiographs. Finally, at Stage 5, end-stage fibrosis of the lungs is noted.

3. d. All of the above. CMV is an opportunistic infection that manifests when a patient's immune system becomes compromised, either by age, medications used to prevent organ rejection, or, more commonly, HIV infection. Although the ocular involvement is the most common form seen in HIV-infected patients, it can affect almost any part of the body, including the GI tract. In the general population, the virus is very common, with about 85% of the U.S. population testing positive for carrying CMV by the time they are 40 years of age.

4. d. Although all of the findings listed can be observed in sarcoid patients, anterior uveitis (granulomatous) is the most frequent ocular finding, reported being seen in up to 55% to 80% of patients during the active stage of the disease. Two types of iris nodules can be observed in sarcoid patients: Koeppe's nodules, which are at the papillary margin, and Busacca's nodules, which are located in the superficial stroma.

5. b. Cidofovir is a virostatic drug approved by the Food and Drug Administration for the treatment of CMV retinitis. It is given intravenously, and its most serious ocular complication is a nongranulomatous uveitis along with hypotony. It can also cause serious, sometimes fatal, systemic problems such as kidney failure or granulocytopenia.

6. d. The ANA test measures the amount of antibodies in patients whose immune system is predisposed to cause inflammation against their own body tissue (i.e., autoantibodies). It is most commonly positive in patients with systemic lupus erythematosus and rheumatoid arthritis, but the test can also be used in the workup for myositis, Sjögren's syndrome, scleroderma, and Hashimoto's thyroid disease.

7. d. After sensitization to a specific allergen, antigen-specific IgE antibodies are created that bind to special receptors located on the surfaces of mast cells and basophils. Then, a reexposure to the antigen results in the antigen binding to and cross-linking the bound IgE antibodies on the mast cells and basophils, which leads to the release of chemical mediators from the mast cells and basophils, causing the signs and symptoms of an immediate hypersensitivity reaction.

8. c. The viral load test measures the amount of HIV virus in blood (copies per milliliter of blood). It can detect the virus within a few days after infection, whereas antibody tests such as ELISA and Western blot can sometimes be negative for months after the initial exposure. Viral load testing is also useful, both for prognosis, where HIV disease progresses quicker in patients with higher viral load, and for managing therapy to assess whether antiviral drugs are being effective.

9. d. With a PPD test, a small amount of protein from TB is injected under the skin. If the person was previously infected with TB, a type IV hypersensitivity (i.e., delayed-type hypersensitivity) reaction mediated by cytotoxic and lymphokine-producing lymphocytes causes an induration at the injection site.

10. c. A normal CD4 count in adults ranges from 500 to 1500 cells per cubic millimeter of blood. The CD4 count typically goes down as HIV disease progresses. Current guidelines recommend that HIV treatment be considered when CD4 count goes below 350. A person who is HIV positive with a CD4 cell count below 200 is diagnosed as having AIDS.

CHAPTER 8

Cardiovascular System

*Albert D. Woods, Greg Black, Julie Tyler,
Michelle Caputo*

CONTENT AREAS

- Epidemiology
- Risk factors for atherosclerotic heart disease
- Coronary artery disease: signs and symptoms
- Significance of palpitations, syncope, murmurs, dyspnea, and claudication
- Pulse and blood pressure: norms, indications, and techniques for evaluation
- Heart failure signs and symptoms
- Laboratory and imaging tests
- Diagnoses and treatment approaches

1. Because the heart fills passively, the circulation rate is normally regulated by:
   a. external temperature
   b. peripheral-vascular factors
   c. cardiac variables
   d. circadian rhythms

2. Common causes of heart failure include all of the following EXCEPT:
   a. incompetent leaky mitral or aortic valves
   b. abnormally slow heart rate secondary to complete heart block
   c. overproduction of thyroid hormones
   d. myocardiopathies of arteriosclerotic, viral, or rheumatic origin

3. Blood pressure is the force of blood:
   a. pushing against the walls of the arteries
   b. traveling through the venous system
   c. being compressed in the left atrium
   d. in the capillary beds

4. Most abnormal pediatric murmurs are due to:
   a. congenital heart disease
   b. cerebral palsy
   c. cystic fibrosis
   d. tachycardia

5. Most abnormal adult murmurs are due to:
   a. stroke
   b. medications
   c. heart valve disease
   d. ventricular arrhythmias

6. What is the leading cause of death in the United States?
   a. stroke
   b. hypertension
   c. diabetes
   d. coronary heart disease

7. High blood pressure affects approximately _____ million people in the United States.
   a. 6.5
   b. 30
   c. 65
   d. 165

8. What class of antihypertensive medications is the preferred first-line therapy for most black and nonblack patients with high blood pressure?
   a. diuretics
   b. beta blockers
   c. calcium channel blockers
   d. alpha-2 agonists

9. The common warning signs of a heart attack may include all the following EXCEPT:
   a. chest and upper body discomfort
   b. shortness of breath
   c. ataxia
   d. cold sweat, nausea, or lightheadedness

10. The common warning signs of cardiac arrest may include all the following EXCEPT:
    a. sudden loss of responsiveness
    b. epistaxis
    c. abnormal breathing
    d. no signs of circulation

11. In the event of cardiac arrest, the first action taken should be to:
    a. initiate CPR (cardiopulmonary resuscitation)
    b. activate an AED (automated external defibrillator)
    c. call 911
    d. perform the Heimlich maneuver

12. Secondary hypertension accounts for what percentage of hypertension?
    a. less than 1%
    b. 5% to 10%
    c. 20% to 25%
    d. 45% to 50%

13. Patients with high blood pressure should avoid or minimize use of all of the following EXCEPT:
    a. cold and flu medications containing decongestants
    b. sodium
    c. physical activity
    d. tobacco

14. Damage to the arterial wall in atherosclerosis is commonly caused by all of the following EXCEPT:
    a. elevated cholesterol/triglyceride levels
    b. tobacco smoke
    c. high blood pressure
    d. diet high in complex carbohydrates

15. Which test uses sound waves to create a detailed, moving picture of the heart?
    a. magnetic resonance imaging (MRI)
    b. echocardiography
    c. electrocardiography (ECG)
    d. coronary angiography

16. One of the most common symptoms of a brain aneurysm is:
    a. dyspnea
    b. claudication
    c. headache
    d. syncope

Answers

1. b. Because there is an association between increased circulation rate and hypertension, most drug therapies for hypertension work to decrease peripheral-vascular resistance, which reduces the circulation rate. The notable exception is diuretic drug therapies, which work by decreasing blood volume, which, in turn, reduces the blood pressure.

2. c. While the overproduction of thyroid hormones will lead to high blood pressure (usually the systolic pressure alone is elevated), along with an increased heart rate, hyperthyroidism is one of the secondary causes of hypertension and rarely leads to heart failure. Secondary causes of hypertension, while uncommon, should always be considered in newly diagnosed or medically nonresponding hypertensive patients.

3. a. Blood pressure is the force of the blood pushing against the walls of the arteries. The systolic pressure is a measurement of the pressure in the arteries as the heart contracts, whereas the diastolic pressure represents the pressure in the arteries as the heart relaxes after a contraction.

4. a. Murmurs are very common in children, and in most cases they are benign and do not indicate heart disease. However, when murmurs are pathologic, congenital heart disease is the leading cause, with an estimated 30,000+ infants born annually with congenital heart defects in the United States.

5. c. Heart valve defects are the most common cause of abnormal murmurs in adults. Although most systolic heart murmurs are benign in adults and are due to increased blood flow velocity, diastolic murmurs and most continuous murmurs usually represent pathologic conditions that require referral for further cardiac evaluation.

6. d. Coronary artery disease occurs when the arteries that supply blood to the heart muscle (i.e., coronary arteries) become hardened and narrowed from plaque buildup, which decreases blood flow and oxygen supply to the heart, leading to coronary heart disease (CHD). It is estimated that more than 13 million people in the United States have some form of CHD.

7. c. High blood pressure affects approximately 65 million adults in the United States, which is about one in every three adults. This is up from 1995, when it was reported that approximately 50 million adults aged 18 and older had high blood pressure. Also, the prevalence increases with age, with more than 50% of those over 60 years of age having some form of hypertension.

8. a. The Antihypertensive and Lipid-Lowering Treatment to Prevent Heart Attack Trial (ALLHAT) study found diuretics to be the best first-line therapy for uncomplicated hypertension.

9. c. Ataxia is lack of coordination caused by dysfunction to sensory nerve inputs or motor nerve outputs or the processing of information between sensory input and motor output. Stroke is an example of a cardiovascular cause of ataxia that occurs when the blood supply to part of the brain is interrupted (i.e., ischemic stroke) or when a blood vessel in the brain ruptures (i.e., hemorrhagic stroke).

10. b. Epistaxis (i.e., nosebleed) can be complicated by hypertension leading to prolonged bleeding, but epistaxis is typically not a sign of cardiovascular compromise or associated with cardiac arrest.

11. c. Call 911 first and then begin CPR immediately. If an AED is available with a trained operator, it can also be used.

12. b. Five to 10 percent of hypertensive patients have an underlying disease that is causing the high blood pressure. Causes of secondary hypertension can include pheochromocytoma, preeclampsia, chronic renal disease, renal artery stenosis, aortic coarctation, hyper- or hypothyroidism, and sleep apnea. The majority of hypertensive patients will have essential or primary hypertension that has no identifiable underlying cause.

13. c. Physical activity can continue. Many over-the-counter cold or flu medications contain decongestants such as pseudoephedrine, phenylephrine, or phenylpropanolamine, which work by constricting blood vessels, causing the blood pressure to elevate. Too much sodium in the diet causes fluid retention, leading to an increase in the overall blood volume, which in turn causes increased blood pressure. Smoking causes narrowing of arteries and also increases the risk of cardiovascular disease; both of these factors lead to faster development of advanced stages of hypertension.

14. d. Diet high in complex carbohydrates. Complex carbohydrates such as vegetables, whole grains, and peas and beans contain various vitamins and minerals, as well as dietary fiber, which all tend to reduce cholesterol levels. Additionally, complex carbohydrates are broken down slowly, which causes a slow increase in insulin levels in contrast to simple carbohydrates (i.e., simple sugars), which break down quickly, increasing the blood sugar levels with an associated insulin surge that promotes the deposition of fat on the vascular endothelium.

15. b. Echocardiography is a noninvasive test that uses ultrasound waves to give either a single-dimension image (M-mode) that allows accurate measurement of the heart chambers or a two-dimensional image to give a cross-sectional view of the beating heart. Coronary angiography is an invasive X-ray examination of the blood vessels or chambers of the heart in which a dye is injected and is typically used to detect obstruction in the coronary arteries. Electrocardiography (ECG) is a noninvasive test that can determine the condition of the heart by recording the electrical activity of the heart. Cardiac MRI is primarily used because of the anatomical detail it provides, including evaluation of aortic dissection, cardiac masses, and congenital heart disease.

16. c. Headache, often described as "the worst headache ever," often occurs with an expanding or ruptured brain aneurysm. It is estimated that 5% of the population has some type of brain aneurysm. However, the incidence of ruptured aneurysms is much lower, at around 0.01% per year in the general population. And in patients who have had one aneurysm, there is a 10% risk of having at least one more.

CHAPTER 9

Renal and Urogenital System

Albert D. Woods, Greg Black, Julie Tyler, Michelle Caputo

1. Blood urea nitrogen (BUN) and creatinine are both used to measure renal function. Which is subject to MORE diurnal variation?
   a. BUN
   b. creatinine
   c. there is no regular diurnal variation with these renal laboratory tests
   d. both have about the same amount of diurnal variation

2. Which of the following does NOT produce polyuria?
   a. diabetes mellitus
   b. rheumatoid arthritis patient on methotrexate
   c. benign prostate hyperplasia (BPH)
   d. diabetes insipidus

3. A urinary tract infection that occurs primarily in the kidney is called:
   a. cystitis
   b. pyelonephritis
   c. glomerulonephritis
   d. urethritis

4. Glomerular filtration rate (GFR):
   a. is a measure of the amount of fluid being filtered by the kidneys in a given amount of time
   b. can be calculated from the concentration of creatinine in a measured urine volume
   c. has no relationship to blood pressure
   d. a, b, and c

5. When using in-office urinalysis reagent strips to test for glucose in urine, positive results usually occur only when:
    a. renal tubules are damaged
    b. blood glucose concentration is above 180 to 200 mg/dL
    c. patient is taking high-dose vitamin C
    d. a and b
    e. a, b, and c

6. All of the following statements regarding renal retinopathy are true EXCEPT:
    a. cotton wool spots are usually very prominent
    b. edema of the retina can be present
    c. blood pressure is usually significantly elevated
    d. optic disc edema may be present

7. All of the following statements regarding Wilms' tumor are true EXCEPT:
    a. children under the age of 5 years with sporadic (i.e., no family history) aniridia are at increased risk of developing Wilms' tumor
    b. chromosome analysis shows a deletion of the short arm of chromosome 11
    c. development of glaucoma is rare in patients with aniridia because there is no iris to block the filtration angle
    d. Wilms' tumor accounts for about 20% of malignant tumors in childhood

8. A positive finding on which of the following urinalysis tests most strongly indicates damage to the renal system?
    a. protein
    b. specific gravity
    d. glucose
    d. ketones

9. Which of the following sexually transmitted diseases has a strong association with pelvic inflammatory disease (PID)?
    a. herpes simplex
    b. gonorrhea
    c. *Chlamydia*
    d. a and b
    e. b and c

10. All of the following are signs of acute renal failure EXCEPT:
    a. edema
    b. high blood pressure
    c. oliguria
    d. broad waxy casts

Answers

1. a. The BUN has a greater diurnal variation than creatinine. Urea is the end product of protein metabolism and is formed in the liver; it then travels via the blood to the kidneys to be excreted in urine. The most common cause of azotemia (elevated BUN) is renal failure or decreased renal function due to compromise in the renal blood supply; however, high-protein diets may also cause abnormally high BUN levels.

2. b. Drugs such as methotrexate, anticholinergics, and diuretics can cause oliguria (decreased urine output), not polyuria. One of the classic symptoms of BPH is polyuria at night because of partial urethra obstruction, which results in incomplete emptying of the bladder. If left untreated, BPH can on rare occasions lead to complete oliguria.

3. b. Pyelonephritis is an infection involving the kidneys. Cystitis, a bladder infection, is seen more frequently than pyelonephritis. Glomerulonephritis is an inflammation of the glomeruli of the kidney. Urethritis is an inflammation of the urethra.

4. a. GFR is the quantity of glomerular filtrate formed each minute by both kidneys and is the best overall indicator of the level of kidney function. GFR can be estimated from formulas that take into account the serum creatinine concentration and other variables such as age, gender, race, and overall body size. Increased blood pressure causes renal afferent arteriolar constriction, which leads to a decreasing GFR.

5. d. Glucose is usually detected in urine only when reabsorbing mechanisms are damaged at the level of the proximal tubules or when the blood glucose concentration exceeds 180 to 200 mg/dL. High doses of vitamin C can cause false-negative results for the amount of glucose in urine when using in-office reagent strips.

6. c. In cases of pure renal retinopathy, the diastolic blood pressure can show only mild to moderate elevation. The retinal findings listed are thought to be secondary to retained nitrogen products due to renal failure and not due to elevated blood pressure.

7. c. Secondary glaucoma develops in almost 50% of patients with aniridia, usually by late childhood. In children where there is a familial history of aniridia, there is no increased risk for developing Wilms' tumor over the general population. However, if there is no family history of aniridia (i.e., sporadic aniridia), there is a greater risk of developing Wilms' tumor.

8. a. With normal kidney function, the larger protein molecules not allowed past the glomerulus and smaller molecules that are filtered by the glomerulus are reabsorbed at the level of the tubules. Thus, finding protein molecules that have passed through the kidney and are in the urine is a sensitive indicator of kidney damage. An abnormal protein urinalysis can be noted months to years before symptoms of renal failure appear. Some medications can cause a small amount of protein to be present with urinalysis testing.

9. e. PID refers to an infection of the fallopian tubes or other internal reproductive organs in women. Female patients with gonorrheal or chlamydial genital infections are at the greatest risk for the development of PID. Untreated PID can lead to infertility, ectopic pregnancy, and chronic pelvic pain.

10. d. Broad waxy casts are typically seen in long-term chronic renal failure and generally indicate a poorer prognosis for the patient. Waxy casts are composed of urinary proteins and other cellular elements entrapped within the cast. Sudden-onset oliguria is the most common and classic finding associated with acute renal failure.

CHAPTER 10

Gastrointestinal System

*Albert D. Woods, Greg Black, Julie Tyler,
Michelle Caputo*

CONTENT AREAS

- Epidemiology
- Common gastrointestinal disorders: signs and symptoms
- Laboratory and imaging tests
- Diagnoses and treatment approaches

1. Four or more large areas of congenital hypertrophy of the retinal pigment epithelium are considered to be a marker for:
   a. ulcerative colitis
   b. Crohn's disease
   c. Whipple's disease
   d. familial polyposis coli
   e. pancreatitis

2. Which of the following gastrointestinal (GI) conditions has a high incidence of premalignant lesions, which requires yearly endoscopy?
   a. cholelithiais
   b. peptic ulcer disease
   c. Barrett's esophagus
   d. *Helicobacter pylori* infection

3. Which medication is used primarily to coat the distal esophagus and stomach contents?
   a. Flagyl
   b. Carafate
   c. Gaviscon
   d. Zantac

4. Up to 90% of patients with gastric or duodenal ulcers that often recur even after healing are found to have _____ colonizing the stomach.
   a. *Helicobacter pylori*
   b. *Enterobacter aerogenes*
   c. Whipple's bacilli
   d. *Lactobacillus acidophilus*

5. You are seeing a patient who is complaining of pain under the right rib radiating to the back and shoulders after eating; the most likely diagnosis is:
    a. peptic ulcer disease
    b. gastroesophageal reflux disease
    c. gallbladder disease
    d. *Helicobacter pylori* infection
    e. Barrett's esophagus

6. All the following are consistent with a diagnosis of Crohn's disease EXCEPT:
    a. perianal sores can be found in up to one third of patients
    b. both the small and large intestine are usually affected
    c. fistulas are common
    d. inflammation of the intestinal mucosa is uniform and continuous
    e. episcleritis can be seen in up to 10% of patients with active disease

7. The GI imaging technique that involves pumping a small amount of air into the lower GI tract and then taking a series of x-rays or CT images that will be used to create a three-dimensional image is:
    a. conventional colonoscopy
    b. virtual colonoscopy
    c. abdominal sonography
    d. electron beam tomography

8. All of the following may be seen in a patient with a malabsorption syndrome EXCEPT:
    a. weight loss
    b. steatorrhea
    c. abdominal indentation (i.e., decreased stomach size)
    d. anemia
    e. diarrhea

1. d. A marker for familial polyposis coli is multiple and bilateral areas of congenital hypertrophy of the retinal pigment epithelium. The retinal lesions often precede the polyposis of the GI tract. The mean age at which colorectal cancer develops from the polyps in these patients is around 39 years and is the leading cause of death.

2. c. Barrett's esophagus is a condition that sometimes develops in patients who have chronic gastroesophageal reflux disease (GERD) or inflammation of the esophagus (esophagitis). Between 5% and 10% of patients with Barrett's esophagus develop cancer in the esophagus. Because of this risk, patients with Barrett's esophagus are screened for esophageal cancer on a regular/yearly basis.

3. c. Gaviscon, an over-the-counter medication, works by coating the surface of the distal esophagus and the surface of stomach contents; this coating prevents acid reflux from damaging the esophagus. Carafate also works by forming a protective coating but is primarily used for the treatment of duodenal ulcers. Although Zantac is used in the treatment of GERD, it is an H_2 blocker, which works to lower the amount of acid produced in the stomach. Flagyl is an antibacterial medication that is sometimes used to treat peptic ulcers but not GERD.

4. a. *Helicobacter pylori* causes more than 80% of gastric ulcers and up to 90% of duodenal ulcers. *H. pylori* is able to survive in the acidic environment of the stomach by living in the mucous lining that also protects the stomach from its own acid. Standard treatment for *H. pylori* includes a combination of two antibiotics and a proton pump inhibitor such as Prilosec.

5. c. The classic symptom of gallbladder disease is sporadic pain in the middle of the upper abdomen or just below the ribs on the right side that can spread to the right shoulder or between the shoulders. There is sometimes associated nausea and vomiting, with the attacks (including the pain aspect) lasting minutes to several hours. Gallbladder disease affects mainly women but can be seen in either sex with GI conditions such as Crohn's disease or ulcerative colitis, obesity, or high blood cholesterol levels.

6. d. One of the key diagnostic findings of Crohn's disease is that while most of the length of the intestine can be involved, the areas of inflammation are very patchy with spots of ulceration with surrounding normal tissue (i.e., skips). The GI ulcers of Crohn's are also more focal and deeper than with ulcerative colitis, with fistulas being common with Crohn's but not seen in ulcerative colitis.

7. b. Virtual colonoscopy is becoming more popular because it does not require the use of a colonoscope, a small flexible tube used to examine the inside of the colon, and imaging quality is much improved over the originally developed x-ray–based systems. With the use of spiral computed tomography, virtual colonoscopy allows a much quicker and more detailed image than do conventional x-rays using a barium enema. On the negative side, virtual colonoscopy does not reveal as much detail as conventional colonoscopy, and tissue samples cannot be taken and polyps cannot be removed during a virtual colonoscopy.

8. c. With malabsorption syndrome, abdominal distention occurs, not abdominal indentation. This distention, or bloating, results from increased intestinal bulk due to material not being absorbed into the body from the digestive tract and from associated gas production. Steatorrhea is an abnormally high amount of fat in the feces due to malabsorption of fat by the intestine and appears as pale, soft, bulky, and malodorous stools.

CHAPTER 11

Liver and Biliary Tract

Albert D. Woods, Greg Black, Julie Tyler,
Michelle Caputo

CONTENT AREAS

- Epidemiology
- Liver and biliary tract disorders: signs and symptoms
- Laboratory and imaging tests
- Diagnoses and treatment approaches

1. All of the following modes of transmission for the different viral hepatitis are correct EXCEPT:
    a. hepatitis B can be spread from mother to child, via sexual intercourse, sharing of contaminated needles, recipient of contaminated blood products, or saliva exposure
    b. hepatitis A is transmitted via the fecal-oral route, mainly by contaminated water, food, or raw shellfish
    c. hepatitis E is usually transmitted from needlesticks, sex, and transfusions
    d. hepatitis C transmission is similar to hepatitis B, except that mother-to-child spread is less common and many patients have no apparent risk factors

2. Which of the following is the most common cause of cirrhosis of the liver worldwide?
    a. chronic alcoholism
    b. hepatitis B
    c. hepatitis C
    d. blocked bile ducts

3. All of the following are consistent with a diagnosis of cirrhosis EXCEPT:
    a. leg edema and ascites
    b. jaundice
    c. itching
    d. weight gain
    e. bruising and bleeding

4. All of the following are risk factors for the formation of gallstones EXCEPT:
    a. high cholesterol levels
    b. male gender
    c. sickle cell anemia
    d. obesity
    e. diabetes

5. Which medication(s) is(are) used for the treatment of chronic hepatitis B?
    a. lamivudine
    b. interferon alfa-2b
    c. adefovir dipivoxil
    d. all of the above

Answers

1. c. Hepatitis E is transmitted in much the same way as hepatitis A, via the fecal-oral route and by contaminated water or food, and is rarely seen in the United States. The only hepatitis not listed was hepatitis D, which is spread similar to hepatitis B, and in humans it occurs only in the presence of a hepatitis B coinfection.

2. b. Hepatitis B infection is the most common cause of cirrhosis worldwide, but it is less common in the United States. In the United States, chronic alcoholism and hepatitis C infection are the most common causes of cirrhosis.

3. d. Patients with cirrhosis lose weight, not gain weight, due in part to a loss of appetite and nausea associated with cirrhosis, as well as to loss of hormonal regulation and cholesterol metabolism that is usually under control of the liver. Ascites is the presence of edema in the peritoneal cavity. Jaundice, a yellowish color noted in the skin and conjunctiva, is from excessive levels of bilirubin. Itching is secondary to bile products being deposited in the skin. Because the liver is involved in the production of proteins needed for blood clotting, cirrhosis causes easy bruising and bleeding and is sometimes noted in the palm of the hands as palmar erythema.

4. b. Females have a higher risk of developing gallstones, not males. In addition to female gender, other conditions that are risk factors for the development of cholesterol gallstones are pregnancy, use of estrogen-containing medications, older age, obesity, high cholesterol levels, and diabetes. Sickle cell anemia is associated with a higher risk of developing pigmented or bilirubin gallstones.

5. d. All of the medications listed can be used in the treatment of hepatitis B. Interferon alfa-2b (Intron A) is given as an injection to help the patient's immune system fight the virus. Lamivudine (Epivir), which was initially developed to treat HIV-infected patients, is also effective against hepatitis B. Adefovir dipivoxil (Hepsera) can help slow the progression of chronic hepatitis B in adults.

CHAPTER 12

Endocrine/Metabolic System

Albert D. Woods, Greg Black, Julie Tyler, Michelle Caputo

CONTENT AREAS

- Epidemiology
- Endocrine disorders: signs and symptoms
- Laboratory and imaging tests
- Diagnoses and treatment approaches

1. Which of the following is NOT a hormone secreted by the pituitary gland?
   a. adrenocorticotropic hormone (ACTH)
   b. follicle-stimulating hormone (FSH)
   c. prolactin
   d. growth hormone
   e. thyrotropin-releasing hormone (TRH)

2. Acromegaly is a disease where there is an excess of which of the following hormones?
   a. ACTH
   b. FSH
   c. prolactin
   d. growth hormone
   e. TRH

3. Which of the following is NOT seen in Addison's disease?
   a. increased pigmentation of the skin
   b. weakness
   c. hypertension
   d. nausea
   e. increased ACTH levels

4. Which of the following visual field defects would you classically expect when a large pituitary tumor has suprasellar extension?
   a. bitemporal hemianopsia
   b. bifrontal hemianopsia
   c. junctional scotoma
   d. central bitemporal scotoma

5. Hypothyroidism is usually characterized by all of the following EXCEPT:
   a. weight gain
   b. heat intolerance
   c. fatigue
   d. dry skin
   e. bradycardia

6. Blood glucose control in diabetics can:
   a. be measured by glycosylated hemoglobin
   b. decrease the incidence of retinopathy if maintained under tight control
   c. require larger doses of insulin for control if insulin resistance is present
   d. a, b, and c

7. Diabetes mellitus is:
   a. diagnosed when the fasting blood glucose is <126 mg/dl
   b. diagnosed when the casual blood glucose is >200 mg/dl
   c. manifested by hypoglycemia
   d. always associated with decreased insulin levels

8. Periorbital myxedema secondary to hypothyroidism is often accompanied by:
   a. blindness
   b. increased facial hair
   c. loss of the lateral third of the eyebrows
   d. photophobia

9. Which of the following is NOT a characteristic of hyperthyroidism?
   a. tachycardia
   b. weight gain
   c. nervousness
   d. pretibial myxedema
   e. tremor

10. In a patient with Cushing's syndrome, which of the following would give the highest level of ACTH?
    a. pituitary tumor
    b. ectopic tumor
    c. adrenal tumor
    d. neither a, b, nor c; ACTH levels are depressed in Cushing's syndrome

11. Which of the following findings is NOT consistent with a diagnosis
of Cushing's syndrome?
    a. deposition of fat on the face and shoulder area
    b. increased incidence of diabetes mellitus
    c. high blood pressure
    d. increased skin pigmentation
    e. elevated IOP

12. In a patient with primary hypothyroidism, the TSH is usually:
    a. elevated
    b. depressed
    c. normal
    d. not used in the diagnosis of hypothyroidism

13. The release of which of the following hormones is directly stimulated
by a decrease in plasma glucose concentrations?
    a. insulin
    b. glucagon
    c. cortisol
    d. growth hormone
    e. none of the above

14. Addison's disease, which is characterized by hypoglycemia and
hyponatremia, reflects a deficit in which hormone(s)?
    a. cortisol
    b. testosterone
    c. glucagon and insulin
    d. cortisol and aldosterone
    e. aldosterone

15. ACTH:
    a. is secreted by the posterior pituitary
    b. secretion is regulated by a hypothalamic secretion
    c. causes the release of hormones from the adrenal medulla
    d. directly stimulates water retention

16. The hormone(s) produced by the kidneys that stimulates the bone
marrow to produce red blood cells is(are):
    a. prostaglandins
    b. levothyroxine
    c. cytokines
    d. erythropoietin

Answers

1. e. Thyrotropin-releasing hormone (TRH) is a neurosecretory hormone released by the hypothalamus; via hypothalamopituitary portal vessels, it goes to the anterior pituitary, where it causes the release of thyroid-stimulating hormone. The other hormones listed are all produced in the anterior pituitary.

2. d. Excess growth hormone, also known as somatotropin, causes acromegaly in adults or giantism when it occurs in children or adolescents. Somatotropin affects growth by playing a part in the metabolism of proteins, fats, and carbohydrates.

3. c. Addison's disease leads to adrenal insufficiency or failure, which causes a slow progressive loss of both cortisol and aldosterone secretion. In particular, aldosterone regulates salt and water levels, which affects both blood volume and blood pressure. Because of the reduced aldosterone, blood pressure is low and falls even further when a person is standing, sometimes producing lightheadedness.

4. a. Bitemporal hemianopsia is the most common visual field loss with suprasellar extension of a pituitary tumor. Because the nasal fibers crossing in the chiasm are compressed from below by the tumor, the first loss is a superior bitemporal hemianopsia, which often progresses to involve both complete temporal hemifields.

5. b. Patients with hypothyroidism have an overall decrease in the body's metabolism rate, which causes a cold intolerance, not a heat intolerance, problem.

6. d. All of the above. Hb_{A1c} test measures the amount of glycosylated hemoglobin, which reflects the average blood glucose level over the past 3 to 4 months. Normal values for a nondiabetic person are 4.0% to 6.0%, with the goal for diabetics to have a value of less than 7.0%. The Diabetes Control and Complications Trial (DCCT) showed that diabetics who maintained blood glucose and glycosylated hemoglobin levels at or close to a normal range decreased their risk of various diabetic complications by 50% to 75%. Up to 90% of type 2 diabetics suffer from insulin resistance, requiring in some patients the starting of insulin injections or increasing the doses in those already on insulin to obtain better control of blood glucose levels.

7. b. Diabetes is diagnosed when the casual (i.e., random) blood glucose is greater than 200 mg/dl; usually the test is repeated on a different day to confirm the diagnosis. In patients with insulin resistance, the pancreas will produce more insulin to attempt to get the glucose out of the blood and into the cells. This leads to hyperinsulinemia, where the blood glucose levels may remain normal for a while, but the high levels of insulin usually cause the person to eat more; this represents an independent risk factor for heart disease and cannot be maintained forever.

8. c. Patients who are hypothyroid often have periorbital myxedema and madarosis, usually the lateral third. Although thyroid ophthalmopathy, as seen in hyperthyroid patients, can occur in patients with hypothyroidism, it is rare. The most common cause of hypothyroidism in the United States is Hashimoto's disease, which is due to a chronic autoimmune thyroiditis.

9. b. Because of the increased metabolism associated with hyperthyroidism, patients usually lose weight even though they may be eating more. Pretibial myxedema, although associated with hyperthyroidism, is a relatively rare finding consisting of a diffuse, nonpitting edema along with thickening of the skin on the anterior aspect of the lower legs that spreads to the dorsum of the feet.

10. b. Cushing's syndrome is characterized by an excess of cortisol, which is usually caused by increased ACTH production. Ectopic tumors usually secrete ACTH and give rise to the highest ACTH levels because they are outside of the normal negative feedback loop. About 15% of Cushing's syndrome cases are secondary to ectopic tumors, with small cell carcinoma of the lung being the most common.

11. d. Increased skin pigmentation is a classic sign associated with Addison's disease, not Cushing's syndrome. It results secondary to adrenal hyposecretion that produces less corticosteroids in the blood; this causes less negative feedback at the level of the pituitary. Hypersecretion of melanocyte-stimulating hormone by the pituitary gland occurs, leading to the formation of excess pigment in the skin and lining of the mouth.

12. a. Scrum TSH (thyroid-stimulating hormone) is the most sensitive test for the diagnosis of primary hypothyroidism, and with no negative feedback controlling an intact pituitary with primary hypothyroidism TSH levels are typically elevated. In contrast, patients with secondary hypothyroidism, where the pituitary gland is not intact, may have low or normal (but with decreased bioactivity) levels of TSH.

13. b. Glucagon mobilizes glucose from its major storage source, liver glycogen, via the process of glycogenolysis, the breakdown of glycogen to glucose, when plasma glucose levels drop.

14. d. Addison's disease results from a severe or total deficiency of the steroid hormones made in the adrenal gland cortex, cortisol and aldosterone. Addison's disease is relatively rare today, with most cases being autoimmune mediated (~70%) or due to TB (~20%), amyloidosis, fungal infection, and adrenalectomy.

15. b. Corticotropin-releasing hormone (CRH) from the hypothalamus acts on the anterior lobe of the pituitary to release ACTH, which travels through the bloodstream to the adrenal cortex. In the adrenal cortex, it initiates the production and release of cortisol and aldosterone. Aldosterone stimulates the kidneys to start the active uptake of sodium (Na^+), which consequently causes the retention of water.

16. d. Erythropoietin is produced in the kidneys and circulates in the blood until it reaches the bone marrow, where it induces red blood cell production, a process known as erythropoiesis. Synthetic erythropoietin is available in the United States as Epogen and Procrit and is used to treat the anemia of cancer chemotherapy, end-stage renal failure, and HIV infection.

CHAPTER 13

Reproductive System

Albert D. Woods, Greg Black, Julie Tyler, Michelle Caputo

1. Women who are pregnant may present with all of the following symptoms EXCEPT:
    a. amenorrhea
    b. decreased urination
    c. tender, swollen breasts
    d. darkening of line from navel to pubis

2. A first-time pregnant female presents reporting swelling of the hands and face and sudden excessive weight gain. Protein is detected in urine testing. This patient most likely has:
    a. premature rupture of the membranes
    b. eclampsia
    c. preeclampsia
    d. ectopic pregnancy

3. Fetal alcohol syndrome (FAS) is a group of serious health problems that develops in the infant of mothers who drink heavily during pregnancy. Babies born with this syndrome may present with the following characteristics:
    a. small eyes and jaws, as well as other possible birth defects
    b. large eyes, overweight, and sleeping excessively
    c. tall and thin due to an anomaly in growth hormones
    d. effects that may be only temporary and resolve after the child is weaned from alcohol addiction

4. Amniocentesis is generally performed between weeks 16 and 18 of pregnancy in order to detect what condition?
    a. Down syndrome and other known hereditary conditions that run in the family
    b. gestational diabetes
    c. group B streptococcal infection
    d. ectopic pregnancy

5. According to the CDC's National Center on Birth Defects and Developmental Disabilities, the incidence of birth defects in the United States is:
   a. 1 in 18
   b. 1 in 33
   c. 1 in 100
   d. 1 in 1500

Answers

1. b. Women who are pregnant generally have more frequent urination starting at about 6 to 8 weeks after conception, not decreased urination. Amenorrhea (the absence of menstruation) generally occurs during the entire pregnancy. Loss of menstrual period can also occur in patients due to travel, stress, significant weight loss or extreme weight gain, and hormonal problems. Tender, swollen breasts can occur as early as a few days after conception and may also be due to birth control pills or premenstrual periods. Darkening of the line between the navel to the pubis occurs during the fourth or fifth month in some pregnant females.

2. c. Preeclampsia (also known as toxemia syndrome or pregnancy-induced hypertension) often begins with the symptoms described along with elevated blood pressure. Premature rupture of the membranes can occur hours to weeks prior to delivery and presents with complaints of leaking fluid, vaginal discharge or bleeding, and pelvic pressure. Eclampsia is the final stage of preeclampsia and is characterized by convulsions or coma. An ectopic pregnancy occurs when a fertilized egg implants outside the uterus, generally in a fallopian tube, and usually presents with pain and tenderness that often start on one side.

3. a. Babies born with FAS may present with facial anomalies, including small eyes and jaws. The infants tend to be overall small in size and have additional birth defects, including heart problems and mental retardation. Due to an anomaly in growth hormones, the children tend to be of short stature and often have learning disabilities. Unfortunately, the effects are not temporary.

4. a. Amniocentesis is generally performed between weeks 16 and 18 of pregnancy to detect Down syndrome and other known hereditary conditions that run in the family and to confirm positive testing results from screening tests. Gestational diabetes may be determined by blood glucose testing (typically occurs around month 5). Group B streptococcal infection may be determined by obtaining a sample from the cervix at 35 to 37 weeks. Ectopic pregnancy is generally confirmed with ultrasound evaluation and on the basis of patient symptoms.

5.   b.   One of every 33 babies in the United States is born with a birth defect. Heart defects are the most common, occurring in about one fourth to one third of all infants born with birth defects. Other common birth defects are "neural tube defects," such as spina bifida, anencephaly, and defects of the lip and roof of the mouth, including cleft lip and cleft palate. While less frequent, there are many hereditary conditions that can lead to birth defects, with Down syndrome being one of most common birth defects.

CHAPTER 14

Respiratory System

Albert D. Woods, Greg Black, Julie Tyler, Michelle Caputo

CONTENT AREAS

- Epidemiology
- Symptoms, signs, and significance of respiratory disorders and anaphylaxis
- Medical laboratory tests, diagnostic imaging, and spirometry
- Diagnoses and treatment approaches

1. Low levels of serum alpha-1 antitrypsin are most strongly associated with which of the following diseases?
   a. sarcoidosis
   b. chronic bronchitis
   c. emphysema
   d. tuberculosis

2. From the following list of standard spirometry abbreviations, which of the measurements represents the volume of air forcefully exhaled in 1 second?
   a. FVC
   b. PEF
   c. FEF_{25-75}
   d. FEV_1

3. All of the following are clinical signs of anaphylaxis EXCEPT:
   a. angioedema
   b. urticaria
   c. spiking blood pressure elevations
   d. rapid pulse
   e. a, b, c, and d

4. Chronic obstructive pulmonary disease (COPD) includes which of the following diseases?
   a. chronic bronchitis
   b. emphysema
   c. asthma
   d. a and b
   e. a, b, c, and d

5. All of the following are common causes of hemoptysis in industrialized countries such as the United States EXCEPT:
   a. bronchitis
   b. aspergillosis
   c. bronchiectasis
   d. bronchogenic carcinoma

6. Which of the following medications used in the treatment of asthma can potentially raise IOP?
   a. montelukast (Singulair)
   b. omalizumab (Xolair)
   c. triamcinolone (Azmacort)
   d. cromolyn (Intal)

7. All of the following statements regarding the Mantoux skin test for tuberculosis (TB) are correct EXCEPT:
   a. measurement is read between 48 and 72 hours after tuberculin injection
   b. measurement is the diameter of the indurated and erythemic area
   c. Mantoux skin test is also called the purified protein derivative (PPD) test
   d. anergy testing is sometimes done with a Mantoux skin test and may include extracts from mumps, *Candida*, or tetanus

8. Which group from the following list has the highest risk of developing COPD?
   a. Hispanics
   b. African Americans
   c. Caucasians
   d. Asians

9. Which of the following statements regarding lung cancer is (are) correct?
   a. it is the leading cancer killer in both men and women in the United States
   b. the majority of lung cancer cases are caused by smoking
   c. males have a higher rate of lung cancer than do females
   d. the 5-year survival rate for patients with lung cancer is lower than that for breast, colon, or prostate cancer
   e. all are true

10. All of the following could be indicated in the management of anaphylaxis EXCEPT:
    a. intramuscular or subcutaneous injection of epinephrine
    b. intravenous atenolol
    c. supplemental oxygen
    d. intravenous hydrocortisone

11.   Sleep apnea has been associated with ocular conditions such as anterior
      ischemic optic neuropathy, papilledema, and floppy lid syndrome. All
      of the following are correct regarding sleep apnea EXCEPT:
      a.   obesity is a predisposing factor
      b.   African Americans have a higher incidence of sleep apnea than do
           Caucasians
      c.   sleep apnea is most commonly due to a neurologic cessation of
           respiratory effort during sleep
      d.   continuous positive airway pressure (CPAP) devices used during
           sleep can be effective in the management of sleep apnea

12.   Which of the following findings is (are) consistent with a diagnosis
      of chronic bronchitis?
      a.   secondary polycythemia
      b.   mucus-producing cough
      d.   elevated lung capacity with a high residual volume
      d.   a and b

13.   An induration of _____ or more millimeters (mm) is considered
      a positive PPD test for a person from the United States with no
      TB risk factors:
      a.   5
      b.   8
      c.   10
      d.   12
      e.   15

14.   The volume of air inhaled and exhaled in a normal breath is
      termed the:
      a.   tidal volume
      b.   vital capacity
      c.   inspiratory capacity
      d.   expiratory reserve volume

15.   All of the following symptoms occurring during respiratory failure are
      due to hypoxemia EXCEPT:
      a.   cyanosis
      b.   hyperventilation
      c.   myoclonus
      d.   seizures

16.   COPD is the ___ leading cause of death in the United States:
      a.   first
      b.   second
      c.   third
      d.   fourth
      e.   fifth

1. c. Emphysema patients have low levels of alpha-1 antitrypsin, which normally protects the lungs from neutrophil elastase. The enzyme neutrophil elastase is released naturally by the lungs to digest damaged cells or bacteria. However, in patients with emphysema, there is insufficient alpha-1 antitrypsin to stop the neutrophil elastase from continuing on and attacking normal lung tissue.

2. d. The FEV_1 (forced expiratory volume in 1 second) is the volume of air that is forcefully exhaled in 1 second. FVC (forced vital capacity) is the maximum volume of air that can be forcefully exhaled, PEF (peak expiratory flow) is the peak flow rate during expiration, and the FEF_{25-75} (forced expiratory flow) is the average forced expiratory flow during the middle (25% to 75%) portion of the FVC.

3. c. During anaphylaxis, there is both decreased vascular tone and capillary leakage, which causes a marked drop in blood pressure leading to anaphylactic shock. It is either the angioedema of the throat and bronchial spasm that leads to obstruction of breathing or the anaphylactic shock that is the major cause of death during anaphylaxis.

4. d. In general, only chronic bronchitis and emphysema are classified as COPD. Even though asthma has an obstructive component, it is usually reversible, so typically asthma is considered a restrictive lung disease, not obstructive. However, studies show that adults with asthma are up to 12 times more likely to develop COPD than are those who do not have asthma.

5. b. Aspergillosis, caused by the fungus *Aspergillus fumigatus*, is a rare cause of hemoptysis (i.e., coughing up blood from the respiratory tract) except in patients who are immunocompromised. Bronchitis is an inflammation of the bronchi and is one of the most common causes of hemoptysis. Bronchiectasis, a chronic dilation and infection of the bronchioles, is another common cause of hemoptysis. Bronchogenic carcinoma, although not as common as bronchitis or bronchiectasis as a cause of hemoptysis, is important because approximately 90% of lung cancers are bronchogenic in origin.

6.   c.   Triamcinolone (Azmacort) is an inhaled corticosteroid that can raise IOP in steroid responders. Although about 5% of the general population will show increased IOP with short-term steroid use, with long-term use, this increases to about 50%, and it is even higher in patients with a family history of glaucoma or patients with diabetes or high myopia. Other common trade name (i.e., brand name) medications used in the treatment of asthma that can increase IOP include Beclovent, Vanceril, Pulmicort, AeroBid, Flovent, Atrovent, and Combivent.

7.   b.   Only the area of induration (i.e., raised area) around the site of the injection is measured; the area of erythema surrounding the indurated area is not measured. Patients with weakened immune systems, such as HIV-infected patients, may not be able to react to the TB skin test. To rule out a false-negative reaction, an anergy panel is typically performed using two substances other than tuberculin, including extracts from mumps, *Candida,* or tetanus. Most people will have a skin reaction to one or more of these extracts.

8.   c.   Caucasians are at the highest risk for the development of COPD. African Americans, Asians, and Hispanics all have both a lower mortality and prevalence rate compared with Caucasians. Interestingly, Asians may have a genetic component that lessens their risk of COPD regardless of smoking habits, one of the greatest risk factors for the development of COPD.

9.   e.   All are correct. Lung cancer kills more people than the next three most common cancers combined (i.e., colon, breast, and prostate cancer). Smoking causes an estimated 87% of all lung cancer cases. Lung cancer is still more common in males, but incidence rates have been decreasing among males while increasing significantly in females. The 5-year survival rate for patients with lung cancer is 15% compared with 63% for colon, 88% for breast, and 99% for prostate cancer.

10.   b.   Atenolol is a beta-blocker, which worsens the signs of anaphylactic attack. Usually patients who are already on a systemic beta-blocker for treatment of a disease and then have anaphylaxis require larger doses of epinephrine, including possible intravenous dosing. Intravenous hydrocortisone is useful in the treatment of bronchospasm and prevention of relapses associated with anaphylaxis.

11. c. The most common form of sleep apnea is obstructive, which is characterized by repetitive pauses in breathing during sleep due to the obstruction and/or collapse of the upper airway. Central sleep apnea, where a neurologic condition causes cessation of respiratory effort during sleep, is much less common. Nasal CPAP devices work by increasing the air pressure in the airways, which keeps the airways from collapsing and creating an obstruction.

12. d. A mild polycythemia may occur secondary to the hypoxia associated with chronic bronchitis. Chronic bronchitis is defined by the presence of the mucus-producing cough being present on most days of the month for at least 3 months of the year and for 2 successive years. Elevated lung capacity with a high residual volume is more commonly associated with emphysema and is due to the breakdown of the walls of the alveoli, which increases overall lung capacity but not respiratory function.

13. e. For a person with no risk factors for TB, 15 mm or more is considered a positive finding. For foreign-born persons in the United States, 10 mm or more is a positive finding, and HIV-infected patients with 5 mm or more induration are considered positive on the PPD. Being positive on the PPD does not mean the person has active disease; additional testing such as chest radiographs, bacteriologic examination, and culturing is needed to determine if active disease is present.

14. a. Tidal volume is the total amount of air that is inhaled and exhaled in a normal breath. The maximum amount of air that can be inhaled and exhaled in a single breath is termed the vital capacity. Inspiratory capacity is the maximal volume inspired starting from a resting expiratory level. Expiratory reserve volume is the maximal amount of air that can be expelled from the lungs after a normal expiration.

15. b. Hyperventilation is usually secondary to the hypercapnia aspect of respiratory failure. Hypercapnia is an abnormally high level of carbon dioxide in the blood. The other findings listed are due to hypoxemia, which is a reduced oxygen level in the blood.

16. d. COPD is the fourth leading cause of death in the United States. Starting in 2000, females have exceeded males in the number of deaths attributable to COPD. It is estimated that more than 11 million adults in the United States have COPD, with more than 120,000 deaths each year from the disease.

CHAPTER 15

Nutrition

Albert D. Woods, Greg Black, Julie Tyler, Michelle Caputo

CONTENT AREAS

- Epidemiology
- Nutritional abnormalities
- Eating disorders
- Medical laboratory testing
- Diagnoses and treatment approaches

1. Which of the following vitamins or supplements is NOT recommended during pregnancy?
   a. folic acid (400 micrograms daily)
   b. high-dose calcium (2 g daily)
   c. high-dose vitamin A (1 million IU daily)
   d. multivitamin (standard dose)

2. All of the following are a sign of vitamin A deficiency EXCEPT:
   a. night blindness
   b. growth retardation
   c. Bitot's spots on the conjunctiva
   d. increased intracranial pressure

3. All of the following are signs of anorexia nervosa EXCEPT:
   a. weight 85% or less than expected based on age and height
   b. cuts and calluses on the back of the hands and knuckles
   c. decreased sex hormones in males
   d. menstrual periods that have stopped in women

4. All of the following can be an impediment to proper nutrition in the elderly EXCEPT:
   a. a good relationship with health care providers
   b. difficulty chewing
   c. alcoholism
   d. loss of appetite

5. Which of the following supplements used in the Age-Related Eye Disease Study (AREDS) may increase the risk of cancer in smokers?
   a. vitamin C
   b. vitamin E
   c. beta-carotene
   d. zinc

6. The laboratory tests directly related to nutrition include all of the following EXCEPT:
    a. testosterone
    b. cholesterol and triglycerides
    c. blood glucose
    d. rapid plasma reagin screening test

Answers

1. c. High-dose vitamin A is associated with birth defects and should not be taken in a high dose during pregnancy. Accutane, used in the treatment of severe acne, has a chemical structure similar to vitamin A and is also known to produce severe birth defects if taken during pregnancy. High-dose calcium can be beneficial due to its ability to decrease maternal blood pressure. Folic acid reduces the risk of neural tube defects, and multivitamins can help reduce the risk of facial clefts.

2. d. Increased intracranial pressure (ICP) is a sign of vitamin A toxicity from too much vitamin A. If the ICP elevates sufficiently (usually greater than 200 to 225 mm H_2O), then clinical signs of pseudotumor cerebri such as swollen optic nerve heads and headache may be present. Bitot's spots are foamy gray or white irregularly shaped patches that appear on the conjunctiva as part of the xerophthalmic (i.e., drying) condition when vitamin A levels are too low. Night blindness is an early manifestation of vitamin A deficiency and is usually noted prior to any xerosis of the conjunctiva.

3. b. Cuts and calluses are associated with bulimia nervosa, in which a person eats in a period of time an amount of food greater than what most people would eat during a similar period of time along with a sense of lack of control over eating during the episode. Inappropriate compensatory behavior in patients with bulimia nervosa to prevent weight gain may include self-induced vomiting; misuse of laxatives, diuretics, and enemas; periods of fasting; and/or excessive exercise or nervous habits. The other findings listed are consistent with anorexia nervosa, in which a person will starve to become very thin due to an intense fear of gaining weight and a distorted body image. Amenorrhea, the absence of at least three consecutive menstrual cycles, is also part of the anorexia disorder.

4. a. A good relationship with health care providers is essential to educating the geriatric population on both health and nutrition. There are many factors that can lead to malnutrition in older adults. A decreased sense of taste or smell; difficulty chewing or swallowing due to poor dentition; chronic diseases and medications that can interfere with appetite, digestion, and absorption of certain nutrients; depression and age-related dementia; and social isolation all can lead to poorer nutrition in the elderly.

5. c. Beta-carotene has been shown to increase the risk of lung cancer among smokers in two different studies. The Alpha Tocopherol Beta Carotene Cancer Prevention Study looked at whether taking alpha tocopherol (vitamin E) and beta carotene daily could reduce the risk of lung cancer; however, 18% more lung cancers developed in persons taking the supplement combination. The Beta Carotene and Retinol Efficacy Trial looked at whether taking beta carotene and retinol (vitamin A) could prevent cancer in smokers and ex-smokers. This study was halted early (~4 years), when it was found that there were 28% more cases of lung cancer diagnosed in those taking the supplements.

6. d. Rapid plasma reagin is a screening test for syphilis, not for determining nutritional status. Low testosterone levels can lead to a decrease in body mass and strength due to loss of muscle tissue and can also cause an increase in body fat. High levels of cholesterol and triglycerides raise the risk of developing heart disease. High blood glucose is associated with a risk of developing diabetes.

CHAPTER 16

Mental Illness and Behavioral Disorders

Albert D. Woods, Greg Black, Julie Tyler, Michelle Caputo

1. According to nationally run studies, the percentage of adults who have a serious mental illness in any year in the United States is:
    a. 2% to 4%
    b. 5% to 7%
    c. 8% to 10%
    d. greater than 10%

2. All of the following are symptoms of schizophrenia EXCEPT:
    a. delusions
    b. hallucinations
    c. heightened affect
    d. trouble concentrating

3. Which of the following can be a sign of child abuse?
    a. subconjunctival hemorrhage
    b. patterned burns
    c. detached retina
    d. bone fractures
    e. a, b, c, and d

4. All of the following are physiologic tests used to help access the presence or degree of mental illness EXCEPT:
    a. Wechsler Memory Scale (WMS-III)
    b. Minnesota Multiphasic Personality Inventory (MMPI-2)
    c. Millon Clinical Multiaxial Inventory (MCMI)
    d. Beck Depression Inventory (BDI)

5. Which of the following drugs is a stimulant that can be made from over-the-counter pseudoephedrine-containing drugs such as Sudafed?
    a. phenobarbital
    b. cocaine
    c. methadone
    d. methamphetamine

Answers

1. b. Between 5% and 7% of adults in the United States have a serious mental illness in any given year. Serious mental illness is defined as a diagnosable mental disorder in persons aged 18 years and older that lasts long enough and is serious enough to interfere with a person's ability to take part in major life activities.

2. c. Patients with schizophrenia typically have a blunted affect with limited facial expressions and emotions. The most common form of hallucination in schizophrenia is auditory (i.e., hearing voices); however, hallucinations can also be visual, olfactory, or felt. Delusions are false ideas that a person has about himself or herself or his or her surroundings.

3. e. Ocular signs of child abuse can occur after either direct trauma or shaking and can involve basically any structure of the eye. Multiple fractures can be observed in 10% to 20% of all abused children. Nonaccidental burns are noted in approximately 10% of all physically abused children and are usually deeper than accidental burns, causing a high degree of scarring and disfigurement.

4. a. The Wechsler Memory Scale (WMS-III) is designed to assess learning, memory, and working memory, not mental illness. The other tests listed can all evaluate different aspects of mental health. The primary focus of the MMPI-2 is identifying pathologic mental illness and disorders. The MCMI was constructed with scales that represented personality disorders and mental illness; however, there is significant debate that this test is not valid across cultural, ethnic, and language barriers. The BDI measures characteristic attitudes and symptoms of depression.

5. d. Methamphetamine is made in illicit laboratories from a mix of around 30 assorted substances, including pseudoephedrine. Methamphetamine gets its effect by causing the release of high levels of dopamine, which is associated with positive emotions. The Substance Abuse and Mental Health Administration reported that 5.7% of all adults over 26 years of age had used the drug in 2004.

CHAPTER 17

Infectious Diseases

Albert D. Woods, Greg Black, Julie Tyler,
Michelle Caputo

1. What percentage of patients with genital gonorrheal infections also present with chlamydial infections?
   a. 0% to 19%
   b. 20% to 39%
   c. 40% to 60%
   d. 65% to 80%

2. Rashes on the palms of the hands and soles of the feet are possible with all of the following EXCEPT:
   a. Lyme disease
   b. erythema multiforme
   c. syphilis infection
   d. pseudoxanthoma elasticum (PXE)

3. According to the World Health Organization, what is the approximate number of people living worldwide with HIV/AIDS following the end of 2004?
   a. 16 million
   b. 27 million
   c. 39 million
   d. 50 million

4. Under the microscope, this condition, which may produce a nontender preauricular node, demonstrates inclusion bodies inside infected host cells.
   a. Neisseria gonorrhoea
   b. herpes simplex virus
   c. cat scratch disease
   d. *Chlamydia trachomatis*

5. In the event of *Toxoplasmosis gondii* infection, appropriate treatment would include a combination of all of the following EXCEPT:
    a. pyrimethamine
    b. sulfadiazine
    c. folinic acid
    d. chloramphenicol

6. What condition is characterized by intensely painful vesicular eruptions on the skin, usually along a dermatome?
    a. herpes simplex virus
    b. herpes zoster virus
    c. Epstein-Barr virus
    d. rubella

7. How are people treated who have a positive PPD and a negative chest x-ray but have been exposed to active TB?
    a. with medicines such as doxycycline
    b. with medicines such as isoniazid (INH)
    c. with no medications
    d. with surgical excision

8. Which of the following laboratory tests for gonorrhea is least invasive?
    a. nucleic acid hybridization tests (e.g., DNA probe test, molecular probe test)
    b. nucleic acid amplification tests (NAATs)
    c. Gram stain
    d. culture

Answers

1. c. *Chlamydia trachomatis* is the most common sexually transmitted disease (STD) in the developed world. It is associated with other STDs with one of the most common being gonorrhoea. Because of the high association of these two STDs occurring together, dual therapy against both is often used even if only one is tested for or diagnosed. In part, because of marked gonococcal resistance to tetracycline, and increasing cases of chlamydial resistance, tetracycline is no longer recommended by the CDC for the treatment of chlamydial infections. Mainstays of treatment for either of these two STDs include either doxycycline or azithromycin.

2. d. Rashes on the palms of the hands and soles of the feet are uncommon but possible with Lyme disease and often occur during the secondary stage of syphilis infections. Erythema multiforme is an acute mucocutaneous hypersensitivity reaction of variable severity that in addition to the ocular complications can have rashes that favor the palms and soles along with the extensor surfaces of extremities and face. While pseudoxanthoma elasticum is associated with skin lesions, it does not typically present on the palms of the hands or soles of the feet.

3. c. At the end of 2004, an estimated 39.4 million people worldwide (37.2 million adults and 2.2 million children younger than 15 years) were living with HIV/AIDS. Approximately two thirds of these people (25 million) live in sub-Saharan Africa, with the next highest percentage (8.2 million) living in Asia and the Pacific.

4. d. *Chlamydia trachomatis* presents with inclusion bodies inside infected host cells. While examination of Giemsa-stained cell scrapings can show the presence of inclusion bodies, it is not as sensitive as other testing methods, such as cultures or nucleic acid probes.

5. d. Although chloramphenicol has a wide spectrum of activity against gram-positive and gram-negative cocci and bacilli, it is not used for the treatment of toxoplasmosis (an obligate intracellular parasite). It is usually reserved for significant infections when other drugs are not as effective or more toxic because of a potentially lethal complication of aplastic anemia.

6. b. In patients with a herpes zoster virus infection, the primary physical finding is a rash following a unilateral dermatomal distribution, which may be erythematous, vesicular, pustular, or crusting in form. Extension of the rash to the tip of the nose indicates involvement of the nasociliary nerve and carries a higher risk for ocular involvement.

7. b. If there has been recent exposure to a TB-infected person, then TB prophylaxis requires taking INH daily for up to 1 year. The PPD can also be positive, with a negative chest x-ray, in individuals from other countries who have received the bCG (bacille Calmette-Guérin) vaccine to prevent TB. However, the vaccine becomes less effective with time and there is no reliable method to distinguish PPD reactions caused by bCG vaccination from those caused by TB infection. These patients, if living in the United States, are also treated if there has been a recent exposure to a TB-infected person. Note that once a PPD is reported as positive, it does not need to be performed again because that person will always have a positive reaction for life.

8. b. Nucleic acid amplification tests (NAATs) have the advantage of being used with urine samples and are also highly sensitive (>90%) for the detection of gonorrhea. NAATs include the polymerase chain reaction (PCR) and ligase chain reaction (LCR) tests. The other tests listed require collecting a sample, usually directly from the cervix or urethra.

CHAPTER 18

Congenital/Hereditary Conditions

Albert D. Woods, Greg Black, Julie Tyler, Michelle Caputo

1. Which of the following conditions is the most common autosomal abnormality, occurring in approximately 1 in 700 live births?
    a. cerebral palsy
    b. Down syndrome
    c. Turner's syndrome
    d. fragile X syndrome

2. Patients with Down syndrome possess many typical ocular findings. Which of the following is NOT associated with Down syndrome?
    a. narrow and upward/outward slanting of the rima palpebrarum
    b. white Brushfield spots arranged in concentric rings
    c. Koeppe nodules of the iris
    d. medial epicanthal folds

3. A triad of cataracts, deafness, and congenital heart disease may occur in infants born to mothers who experienced what condition during pregnancy?
    a. rubella
    b. cytomegalovirus (CMV) infection
    c. toxoplasmosis
    d. histoplasmosis

4. Radiologic manifestations of skeletal anomalies in fetal alcohol syndrome include all following EXCEPT:
    a. Klippel-Feil syndrome
    b. hemivertebrae
    c. microcephaly
    d. shortened fifth digits

5. What is the most common lethal inherited disease in Caucasians?
   a. Down syndrome
   b. cystic fibrosis (CF)
   c. toxoplasmosis
   d. retinitis pigmentosis

Answers

1. b. Down syndrome is the most common autosomal abnormality, with three different cytogenic variants: trisomy 21 (accounting for 95%), chromosomal translocation, and mosaicism. Cerebral palsy has a variety of etiologies that may involve problems during development, delivery, or after delivery but not following an autosomal pattern. Turner syndrome is characterized by a short stature and lack of sexual development at puberty. Fragile X syndrome is the most common cause of inherited mental impairment; it is sex-linked with a prevalence of approximately 1 in 3500.

2. c. Koeppe nodules are associated with a granulomatous anterior uveitis, with the nodules being located along the pupillary margin. All of the other findings are associated with Down syndrome, including 80% of patients with the condition having a narrow and upward/outward slanting of the rima palpebrarum, 60% of patients with white Brushfield spots arranged in concentric rings on the periphery of the iris, and, commonly, medial epicanthal folds.

3. a. Rubella can cause a triad of cataracts, deafness, and congenital heart disease in infants born to mothers who experienced rubella during pregnancy. Cytomegalovirus has emerged as an important cause of congenital infection in the developed world, which can lead to mental retardation and developmental disability but not the triad described in the question. Congenital toxoplasmosis infection is seen as a clinical triad of retinochoroiditis, cerebral calcifications, and convulsions. Although histoplasmosis infection is associated with an ocular triad in adults, it does not present congenitally in the described manner.

4. c. Microcephaly is a neurologic finding in which the circumference of the head is smaller than normal because the brain has not developed fully. Klippel-Feil syndrome is a rare disorder where there is a congenital fusion of any two of the seven cervical vertebrae. Hemivertebrae is a congenital partial formation of a vertebra and is most common in the thoracic region.

5. b. Cystic fibrosis is the most common lethal inherited disease in Caucasians. It is an autosomal recessive disorder affecting exocrine gland function, involving multiple organ systems, and resulting in chronic respiratory infections. End-stage lung disease is the principal cause of death, with the median age of survival in the mid-30s.

Part 1 Recommended Reading

Books

Blaustein BH, ed: *Ocular manifestations of systemic disease,* New York, 1994, Churchill Livingstone.

Gold DH, Weingeist TA, eds: *Color atlas of the eye in systemic disease,* Philadelphia, 2001, Lippincott Williams & Wilkins.

Gold DH, Weingeist TA, eds: *The eye in systemic disease,* Philadelphia, 1990, JB Lippincott.

Kanski JJ: *Clinical ophthalmology: a systematic approach,* ed 5, New York, 2003, Elsevier, Health Sciences Division.

Kanski JJ: *Clinical ophthalmology: a test yourself atlas,* ed 2, New York, 2002, Elsevier, Health Sciences Division.

Ostler HB, et al: *Diseases of the eye and skin: a color atlas,* Philadelphia, 2004, Lippincott, Williams & Wilkins.

Regenbogen LS, Eliahou HE, eds: *Diseases affecting the eye and the kidney,* New York, 1993, S. Karger (USA).

Thomann KH, Marks ES, Adamczyk DT, eds: *Primary eyecare in systemic disease,* ed 2, New York, 2001, McGraw-Hill.

Watson PG, et al: *The sclera and systemic disorders,* ed 2, Boston, 2004, Butterworth-Heinemann.

Internet

www.emedicine.com

www.merck.com/mrkshared/mmanual/home.jsp

www.medicinenet.com

www.labtestsonline.org

www.nlm.nih.gov/medlineplus

www.cdc.gov

www.americanheart.org

Ocular Disease and Trauma

CHAPTER 19

Orbit, Adnexa, Lacrimal System

Daniel K. Roberts, Jennifer A. Palombi, Brad M. Sutton

CONTENT AREAS

- Epidemiology and history
- Signs and symptoms
- Techniques and skills
- Pathophysiology and diagnosis
- Treatment, management, and prognosis

1. Orbital cellulitis is most likely to be associated with:
   a. conjunctivitis
   b. chalazion
   c. sinusitis
   d. blepharitis
   e. meningitis

2. Which of the following is NOT a distinguishing feature in the differential diagnosis between preseptal cellulitis and orbital cellulitis?
   a. proptosis
   b. loss of vision
   c. extraocular movements
   d. lid edema

3. Which of the following is a diagnosis of exclusion in the assessment of orbital proptosis?
   a. orbital cellulitis
   b. Graves' ophthalmopathy
   c. pseudotumor cerebri
   d. enophthalmos of the fellow eye
   e. orbital tumor or mass

4. Inflammatory orbital pseudotumor can lead to all of the following EXCEPT:
   a. choroidal folds
   b. proptosis
   c. restriction of ocular motility
   d. myopic refractive error shift

5. A 39-year-old woman presents with painless eyelid edema, bilateral proptosis, and conjunctival injection overlying the horizontal rectus muscle tendons. The patient MOST likely has:
    a. carotid cavernous sinus fistula
    b. Graves' disease
    c. Tolosa-Hunt syndrome
    d. orbital myositis

6. Dacryoadenitis is an inflammation of the _____ and is usually a _____ condition.
    a. lacrimal sac, bilateral
    b. lacrimal gland, bilateral
    c. lacrimal sac, unilateral
    d. lacrimal gland, unilateral

7. Profound loss of vision and afferent papillary defect associated with thyroid orbitopathy are usually the result of:
    a. exposure keratitis
    b. compressive optic neuropathy
    c. lid inflammation
    d. secondary uveitis
    e. chronic dry eye

8. The most common cause of upper eyelid retraction is:
    a. trauma
    b. thyroid ophthalmopathy
    c. inflammatory pseudotumor
    d. Parinaud's syndrome
    e. third nerve palsy with aberrant regeneration

9. Floppy eyelid syndrome is most commonly seen in:
    a. diabetics
    b. elderly females
    c. obese or significantly overweight patients
    d. patients with myasthenia gravis

10. A slowly enlarging, noninflammatory mass that may erode the bony walls of the sinuses and is composed of mucoid and epithelial debris is MOST likely a(an):
    a. dermoid cyst
    b. orbital pseudotumor
    c. cavernous hemangioma
    d. mucocele

11. The reference points for exophthalmometry measurements are
the _____ and the _____.
a. nasal orbital rim, corneal apex
b. outer canthus, limbus
c. outer canthus, corneal apex
d. temporal orbital rim, limbus
e. temporal orbital rim, corneal apex

12. A 29-year-old man presents with a history of orbital medial wall
fracture and possible sixth nerve palsy. A useful test in determining
whether his limitation in lateral gaze is paralytic or the result of muscle
entrapment would be:
a. visual evoked potential
b. forced duction testing
c. palpation of the orbit and globe
d. exophthalmometry
e. cover test

13. A 64-year-old woman has a left lower lid ectropian as a surgical
complication after the removal of a basal cell carcinoma. This
ectropian would be classified as being _____ in nature.
a. cicatricial
b. congenital
c. tarsal
d. paralytic
e. involutional

14. The natural course of a capillary hemangioma in a child is USUALLY
characterized by:
a. complete resolution
b. gradual enlargement requiring excision
c. ulceration, necrosis, and infection
d. malignant transformation

15. Patients with floppy eyelid syndrome experience what type of
symptoms?
a. blurred vision late in the day
b. burning and foreign body sensation that worsens as the day goes on
c. burning and foreign body sensation that improves as the day goes on
d. extreme photophobia

16. An acquired condition in which eyelashes are misdirected toward the
cornea or conjunctiva is:
a. blepharitis
b. trachoma
c. trichiasis
d. entropion

17. All of the following can result in eyelid ptosis EXCEPT:
    a. Marcus-Gunn (jaw wink) phenomenon
    b. third nerve palsy
    c. Horner's syndrome
    d. thyroid orbitopathy
    e. ocular myasthenia

18. Profound dermatochalasis is most likely to have an adverse effect on the results of which of these clinical tests?
    a. pachymetry
    b. applanation tonometry
    c. visual field testing
    d. biomicroscopy
    e. fundoscopy

19. Dacryoadenitis can be caused by all of the following EXCEPT:
    a. sarcoidosis
    b. bacterial infection
    c. viral infection
    d. histoplasmosis

20. Orbital blowout fractures typically affect the _____ of the orbit and result in an apparent _____.
    a. roof, enophthalmos
    b. floor, enophthalmos
    c. floor, exophthalmos
    d. medial wall, exophthalmos
    e. medial wall, enophthalmos

21. The primary treatment for an orbital floor fracture that is resulting in pronounced diplopia and enophthalmos is:
    a. surgical repair of the orbital floor using bone grafts or synthetic material
    b. oral corticosteroid therapy
    c. nonsteroidal anti-inflammatory therapy
    d. observation

22. Congenital nasolacrimal duct obstruction USUALLY requires:
    a. dacryocystorhinostomy (DCR)
    b. lacrimal probing
    c. observation only
    d. oral antibiotic therapy

23. Sudden onset of pain and swelling over the medial canthus that is associated with epiphora is MOST likely to be:
    a. acute dacryocystitis
    b. angular conjunctivitis
    c. dry eye syndrome
    d. staphylococcal blepharokeratoconjunctivitis

24. Which of the following refers to removal of the globe, while leaving the remaining contents of the orbit intact?
    a. evisceration
    b. exenteration
    c. enucleation
    d. exoneration

25. Floppy eyelid syndrome is often associated with:
    a. surgical trauma
    b. sleep apnea
    c. autoimmune disease
    d. Graves' disease
    e. Stevens-Johnson syndrome

26. Which of the following oral antibiotics are appropriate for the treatment of dacryocystitis?
    a. Keflex (cephalexin)
    b. dicloxacillin
    c. doxycycline
    d. a, b, and c
    e. a and b

27. The most common epithelial malignancy of the lid is _____.
    a. malignant melanoma
    b. squamous cell carcinoma
    c. basal cell carcinoma
    d. rhabdomyosarcoma

28. A molluscum contagiosum lesion of the eyelid is the result of:
    a. viral infection
    b. bacterial infection
    c. metastatic disease
    d. meibomianitis
    e. blepharitis

29. During administration of the primary Jones dye test, dye is recovered following the application of a cotton-tipped applicator under the inferior turbinate. This MOST likely indicates:
    a. complete obstruction of the lacrimal drainage system
    b. tearing due to primary hypersecretion
    c. partial obstruction of the lacrimal drainage system
    d. poor function of the valve of Hasner

30. A generalized inflammation of the eyelid anterior to the orbital septum is a(an):
    a. chalazion
    b. hordeolum
    c. primary meibomianitis
    d. preseptal cellulitis

31. Verrucae are caused by:
    a. papillomavirus
    b. *Staphylococcus aureus*
    c. *Haemophilus influenzae*
    d. herpes simplex virus

32. Ocular contact dermatitis is a(an) _____ of the skin around the eye.
    a. infection
    b. allergic reaction
    c. neoplasm
    d. traumatic injury
    e. idiopathic inflammation

33. Which of the following antibiotics would be an appropriate treatment for Meibomian gland dysfunction?
    a. doxycycline
    b. Augmentin
    c. dicloxacillin
    d. Keflex (cephalosporin)

34. Which of the following is most useful in measuring tear production?
    a. dye disappearance test
    b. intracanalicular probing
    c. Jones test
    d. Schirmer's test
    e. irrigation of lower canaliculus

35. Epiphora refers to symptoms of excess tearing due to _____.
    a. lacrimal outflow deficiency
    b. excess production of tears
    c. ocular irritation
    d. age

36. If pressure on the lacrimal sac results in an outflow of mucus from the puncta, the patient most likely has:
    a. dacryoadenitis
    b. dacryocystitis
    c. internal hordeolum
    d. meibomianitis
    e. chronic dry eye

37. What is dacryoadenitis?
    a. infection/inflammation of the lacrimal sac
    b. infection/inflammation of the lacrimal gland
    c. infection/inflammation of the canaliculus
    d. swelling of the lacrimal sac

38. The most common symptom of a disorder in the function or anatomy of the lacrimal drainage system is:
    a. pain
    b. mucus discharge
    c. tearing
    d. photophobia
    e. asthenopia

39. Xanthelasmas are frequently associated with what systemic disorder?
    a. leukemia
    b. non-Hodgkin's lymphoma
    c. hyperlipidemia
    d. coronary artery disease
    e. acne rosacea

40. Marcus-Gunn jaw winking phenomenon is the clinical result of aberrant connections between which two cranial nerves?
    a. CN V and CN III
    b. CN VII and CN III
    c. CN VII and CN V
    d. CN VI and CN VII
    e. CN VI and CN V

41. Which of the following is not an appropriate management option for dacryocystitis?
    a. oral antibiotics
    b. warm compresses with massage
    c. topical antibiotics
    d. dilation and irrigation of the puncta and lacrimal system

42. Orbital bruits are most likely to be associated with:
    a. temporal arteritis
    b. orbital hemangioma
    c. orbital blowout fracture
    d. cavernous sinus fistula

43. Actinic keratoses:
    a. may be a precursor to squamous cell carcinoma
    b. always require surgical removal
    c. have a smooth, waxy surface
    d. are not usually found on sun-exposed regions of the skin

44. Chronic papillary conjunctivitis that is associated with a pliable, rubbery tarsus is MOST likely:
    a. spastic ectropion
    b. floppy eyelid syndrome
    c. myokymia
    d. primary eyelid hypoplasia

45. The most common type of skin cancer in the United States, which also accounts for the majority of malignant eyelid tumors, is:
    a. Kaposi's sarcoma
    b. squamous cell carcinoma
    c. basal cell carcinoma
    d. keratoacanthoma

46. Distichiasis is defined as:
    a. an absence of eye lashes
    b. the loss of eyelashes due to a metastatic lid lesion
    c. an abnormal row of lashes growing from the Meibomian glands
    d. crusting of the eyelashes associated with blepharitis

47. Which of the following oral medications would be most appropriate for treating a child with dacryocystitis?
    a. tetracycline
    b. oral prednisone
    c. amoxicillin
    d. vancomycin
    e. acyclovir

48. What type of lid lesion should be considered in a case of a 45-year-old man with recurrent, unilateral blepharitis and chalazion with an associated loss of eyelashes?
    a. sebaceous gland carcinoma
    b. molluscum contagiosum
    c. basal cell carcinoma
    d. actinic keratosis
    e. xanthelasma

49. A 46-year-old woman presents with complaints of ocular irritation, dryness, and redness. Telangiectasia of the facial blood vessels and facial erythema are noted on gross examination of the adnexa. The likely underlying cause of her ocular discomfort is:
    a. systemic lupus erythematosus
    b. acne rosacea
    c. herpes zoster
    d. Graves' disease
    e. herpes simplex

50. Appropriate long-term therapy for severe, chronic dry eye might include:
    a. topical prednisolone acetate
    b. topical gentamicin
    c. oral prednisone
    d. Vigamox
    e. topical cyclosporine

51. Xanthelasmas are more commonly found in adults with:
    a. hyperlipidemia
    b. hypertension
    c. neurofibromatosis
    d. a history of alcohol abuse

52. Oral acyclovir is MOST effective for herpes zoster ophthalmicus if it is administered within:
    a. 48 to 72 hours after the appearance of the lid lesions
    b. 4 to 5 days after the appearance of the lid lesions
    c. 1 week after the appearance of the lid lesions
    d. 1 month after the appearance of the lid lesions

53. Orbital cellulitis, which may be characterized by the acute onset of unilateral proptosis and chemosis, and painful diplopia:
    a. is an ocular emergency
    b. is treated with topical antibiotics
    c. is not vision threatening
    d. never requires surgical intervention

54. Molluscum contagiosum may:
     a. undergo malignant transformation
     b. result from a cyst of Moll
     c. cause follicular conjunctivitis
     d. cause an iridocyclitis

55. An inability to fully close one eye is frequently caused by which
     of the following?
     a. third nerve palsy
     b. abducens (sixth nerve) palsy
     c. Bell's (seventh or facial) nerve palsy
     d. diabetes

56. The outer layer of the tear film is composed of _____ and
     originates primarily from the _____ of the lids.
     a. mucin, goblet cells
     b. lipid, goblet cells
     c. mucin, Meibomian glands
     d. lipid, Meibomian glands
     e. aqueous, lacrimal gland

57. What condition commonly presents with a classic triad of dry eyes, dry
     mouth, and arthralgia?
     a. rosacea
     b. Sjögren's syndrome
     c. Stevens-Johnson syndrome
     d. keratoconjunctivitis sicca
     e. ocular pemphygoid

58. Evaporative loss of aqueous tears is associated with dysfunction of the
     _____.
     a. lipid tear layer
     b. mucin tear layer
     c. lacrimal gland
     d. lacrimal drainage system

59. Which of the following can be signs or symptoms of an orbital blowout
     fracture?
     a. diplopia
     b. enophthalmos
     c. restriction of ocular motility
     d. a, b, and c

60. A normal tear breakup time is considered to be:
    a. <10 seconds
    b. >10 seconds
    c. >5 seconds
    d. 8 to 12 seconds

Answers

1. c. Orbital cellulitis is most commonly caused by the spread of infection from the paranasal sinuses. The remaining three choices are commonly associated with preseptal cellulitis, a different condition.

2. d. Eyelid edema will occur in both preseptal cellulitis and orbital cellulitis. Proptosis, decreased vision, and limited extraocular movement are distinct to orbital cellulitis and therefore useful in differential diagnosis.

3. c. Orbital cellulitis, enophthalmos, lacrimal gland tumor, and Graves' ophthalmopathy can all be diagnosed with laboratory studies and/ or clinical imaging. Pseudotumor is diagnosed only when no underlying systemic or local cause can be identified.

4. d. Inflammatory orbital pseudotumor is not associated with a myopic shift but is associated with each of the other choices.

5. b. Graves' disease is the only condition that would likely be bilateral. The age and gender of the patient are classic for Graves' disease. Injection overlying the horizontal rectus muscles is also a classic sign.

6. d. Dacryoadenitis is an inflammation of the lacrimal gland and usually presents as a unilateral condition.

7. b. Loss of vision associated with Graves' ophthalmopathy most often results from compression of the optic nerve within the orbit, that is, compressive optic neuropathy.

8. b. While all of these conditions may cause upper lid retraction or the appearance of upper lid retraction, thyroid orbitopathy is the most common cause of upper eyelid retraction.

9. c. Floppy eyelid syndrome is the result of a rubbery tarsal plate and is almost always found in overweight individuals.

10. d. A rhabdomyosarcoma is a malignant orbital tumor not composed primarily of mucoid and epithelial debris. Orbital pseudotumor is an inflammatory tumor. A cavernous hemangioma is a vascular tumor.

11. e. In all exophthalmometry measurements, the primary reference points are the temporal orbital rim posteriorly and the corneal apex anteriorly.

12. b. Forced duction testing is used to differentiate between paralytic muscle underaction and extraocular muscle entrapment.

13. a. Cicatricial ectropian is defined as ectropian caused by shortening of the anterior lamella of the eyelid, most frequently as a result of lid surgery.

14. a. About 75% of capillary hemangioma cases spontaneously involute by age 7.

15. c. The burning, stinging, redness, and foreign body sensation associated with floppy eyelid syndrome improve as the day goes on because the problem occurs when the eyelid spontaneously everts during sleep.

16. c. Trichiasis is an acquired condition in which eyelashes are misdirected posteriorly toward the conjunctiva or cornea. Entropion is an inward misdirection of the entire lid.

17. d. Thyroid orbitopathy causes eyelid retraction, while all other listed conditions result in lid ptosis.

18. c. Dermatochalasis can cause a false superior arcuate defect in visual field testing.

19. d. Histoplasmosis is not associated with dacryoadenitis.

20. b. Orbital blowout fractures typically refer to fractures of the floor of the orbit and result in an apparent enophthalmos due to prolapse of tissue into the fracture.

21. a. Although observation and anti-inflammatory therapy may be indicated, resolution of a significant orbital floor fracture will not occur without surgical intervention.

22. c. Lacrimal probing and DCR are measures required only for persistent duct obstruction. Most cases of congenital duct obstruction will spontaneously become patent within the first few weeks of life.

23. a. Angular conjunctivitis, dry eye syndrome, and staphylococcal blepharokeratoconjunctivitis would not be as likely as dacryocystitis to cause both medial canthal pain and epiphora.

24.   c.   Enucleation is defined as the surgical removal of the entire globe and its contents, while leaving the remaining orbital contents, including the extraocular muscles, intact.

25.   b.   Floppy eyelid syndrome is often found in overweight males with associated sleep apnea.

26.   e.   Keflex and dicloxacillin are excellent choices for the treatment of dacryocystitis, but doxycycline is not potent enough for the treatment of soft tissue infections. There also is too much staphylococcal resistance to doxycycline.

27.   c.   Basal cell carcinoma is the most common epithelial malignancy of the eyelid.

28.   a.   Molluscum contagiosum lesions are benign neoplasms caused by the molluscum contagiosum virus (MCV).

29.   b.   Complete obstruction or partial obstruction of the lacrimal drainage system would not yield the flow of fluorescein dye into the inferior turbinate region. The valve of Hasner would likely be functioning properly if dye traversed the nasolacrimal system to be recovered in the inferior turbinate region.

30.   d.   A chalazion is a focal granuloma of a Meibomian gland, a hordeolum is a localized infection of a sebaceous gland of the lid, and meibomianitis is characterized by a generalized blockage of the Meibomian glands.

31.   a.   Verrucae (warts) are viral in nature. Herpes simplex does not cause lid lesions similar to papillomavirus.

32.   b.   Contact dermatitis is a type 4 immunologic reaction to an allergen.

33.   a.   Only doxycycline among the agents on this list has the ability to alter glandular secretions and improve glandular function.

34.   d.   All of these tests may be used in the evaluation of epiphora, but Schirmer's test is the only one of these aimed at measuring tear production. The others seek to evaluate or facilitate lacrimal outflow.

35.   a.   Epiphora refers to tearing as a result of lacrimal outflow deficiency. Excess production of tears is known as hyperlacrimation.

36. b. Dacryocystitis is an infection of the lacrimal sac. Regurgitation of mucus from the puncta with digital pressure on the lacrimal sac is a common clinical sign.

37. b. Dacryoadenitis involves the lacrimal gland.

38. c. The most common symptom of a disorder in the function or anatomy of the lacrimal drainage system is tearing.

39. c. Xanthelasmas are frequently found in patients with hereditary hyperlipidemia.

40. a. Marcus-Gunn jaw winking syndrome is the result of aberrant connections between the motor branches of the fifth cranial nerve and the superior division of the oculomotor nerve (CN III).

41. d. It is inappropriate to dilate and irrigate the lacrimal system in the presence of active infection of the lacrimal sac because the infection may spread to the throat. Each of the other answers may have a place in the management of dacryocystitis.

42. d. Orbital bruits are detected on auscultation and are generally associated with high-pressure/high-flow cavernous sinus fistulas.

43. a. Actinic keratoses are usually benign but may be a precursor to squamous cell carcinoma up to 25% of the time. They are crusty lesions that may bleed. They can be monitored carefully, although there is malignant potential.

44. b. A rubbery, pliable eyelid is a classic feature of floppy eyelid syndrome. Myokymia is characterized by muscle twitching. Spastic entropion would not be characterized by a rubbery eyelid. Primary eyelid hypoplasia is a fictional term.

45. c. Keratoacanthoma is a benign lesion that can be mistaken for basal cell carcinoma and squamous cell carcinoma. Basal cell carcinomas account for about 90% of all malignant eyelid tumors. Kaposi's sarcoma is much less common than basal cell carcinoma and is usually associated with AIDS.

46. c. Distichiasis is defined as an abnormal row of lashes emanating from the Meibomian glands.

47. c. Amoxicillin is an antibiotic approved for use in children.
         Prednisone is inappropriate therapy for dacryocystitis; vancomycin
         and tetracycline are inappropriate for pediatric use, and acyclovir is
         an antiviral medication (not indicated for dacryocystitis).

48. a. Sebaceous gland carcinoma usually occurs in middle-aged
         (or older) men with a history of unilateral, recurrent blepharitis,
         and/or chalazion. There is a loss of eyelashes and destruction
         of the Meibomian gland orifices at the site of the tumor.

49. b. Acne rosacea presents clinically with telangiectasia of the facial
         blood vessels and facial erythema and may have associated papules
         and/or pustules. The common ocular complication of rosacea
         (ocular rosacea) is chronic dry eye with redness, burning, and
         discomfort.

50. e. Topical cyclosporine is an appropriate and effective long-term
         treatment for chronic dry eye syndrome. Steroids (oral or topical)
         are not appropriate for the long term due to adverse effects, and
         antibiotics are helpful only in cases of infectious processes, such as
         blepharitis.

51. a. Hypertension, neurofibromatosis, and alcohol use are not known
         risk factors for xanthelasma.

52. a. The effectiveness of oral acyclovir for herpes zoster ophthalmicus
         may be substantially reduced or ineffective if not administered
         within 48 to 72 hours of the appearance of the skin lesions.

53. a. Orbital cellulitis is a serious condition requiring immediate
         attention. Intracranial complications such as meningitis, brain
         abscess, and cavernous sinus thrombosis are potential
         complications.

54. c. Molluscum contagiosum are benign lesions caused by one of the
         pox viruses. They are not associated with cysts of Moll and do not
         cause iridocyclitis.

55. c. Bell's palsy leads to the inability to close one eye while none of the
         other potential answers have this result.

56. d. The outer layer is composed of lipid and originates primarily from
         the Meibomian glands of the lids.

57. b. Sjögren's syndrome classically consists of the triad of dry eyes, dry
         mouth, and arthralgia.

58. a. Evaporative loss of aqueous tears is associated with dysfunction of the lipid layer. The outermost lipid layer is responsible for preventing aqueous evaporation.

59. d. All of these findings can be associated with a blowout fracture of the orbit.

60. b. A tear breakup time of greater than 10 seconds is considered to be normal.

CHAPTER 20

Cornea/External Disease

Jennifer A. Palombi, Daniel K. Roberts,
Brad M. Sutton, Leo P. Semes

CONTENT AREAS

- Epidemiology and history
- Signs and symptoms
- Techniques and skills
- Pathophysiology and diagnosis
- Treatment, management, and prognosis

1. Corneal ulceration always begins with:
   a. an epithelial defect
   b. contact lens wear
   c. a primary infection
   d. stromal haze

2. Corneal epithelial microcysts are the physiologic result of:
   a. the mechanical rubbing of a contact lens on the cornea
   b. chronic corneal hypoxia
   c. topical drug toxicity
   d. recurrent corneal erosion

3. A 29-year-old contact lens patient presents with a new corneal lesion that is peripheral, painless, with mild staining and has no associated anterior chamber inflammation. Of the following, the lesion is MOST likely a(an):
   a. infectious corneal ulcer
   b. *Acanthamoeba* infection
   c. sterile infiltrate
   d. corneal microcyst
   e. corneal scar

4. All of the following would be an appropriate therapy for a corneal abrasion EXCEPT:
   a. bandage contact lens
   b. topical antibiotic
   c. oral NSAID
   d. topical steroid

5. Corneal guttata are associated with:
   a. Fuchs' endothelial dystrophy
   b. Map-dot-fingerprint dystrophy
   c. anterior uveitis
   d. recurrent corneal erosion
   e. filamentary keratitis

6. Corneal guttata are an abnormality of:
   a. the corneal stroma
   b. the corneal epithelium
   c. Bowman's layer
   d. Descemet's membrane

7. Which of the following corneal dystrophies is NOT an epithelial dystrophy?
   a. ABMD
   b. Meesman's
   c. Reis-Buckler's
   d. granular

8. Which of the following is NOT a stromal dystrophy of the cornea?
   a. macular dystrophy
   b. granular dystrophy
   c. map-dot-fingerprint dystrophy
   d. lattice dystrophy

9. All of the following are characteristic of corneal dystrophies EXCEPT:
   a. unilateral
   b. genetically inherited
   c. progressive
   d. not associated with systemic or local disease

10. The "dots" in map-dot-fingerprint corneal dystrophy are:
    a. guttata
    b. folds in Descemet's membrane
    c. intraepithelial microcysts
    d. corneal scars

11. Dermatoses and hypersensitivities can mimic neoplasia of the lids, for example. The most common eruption of the eyelids is:
    a. contact dermatitis
    b. psoriasis
    c. rosacea
    d. lichen planus

12. A dendritic corneal ulcer is a classic presentation of:
     a. herpes zoster
     b. *Pseudomonas aeruginosa*
     c. herpes simplex
     d. *Candida albicans*

13. All of the following may be used in the initial treatment of herpes
     simplex keratitis EXCEPT:
     a. trifluridine gtts
     b. oral acyclovir
     c. homatropine gtts
     d. prednisolone acetate gtts
     e. vidarabine ung

14. The leading systemic cause of interstitial keratitis is:
     a. syphilis
     b. herpes zoster
     c. acne rosacea
     d. lupus

15. Which of the following corneal dystrophies is NOT a stromal
     dystrophy?
     a. posterior polymorphous dystrophy
     b. macular
     c. avellino
     d. lattice

16. Keratoconjunctivitis sicca is the direct result of:
     a. staphylococcal toxicity
     b. inadequate tear film protection
     c. contact lens–induced corneal hypoxia
     d. lagophthalmos

17. On examination, a 32-year-old man demonstrates an increase in
     myopia and astigmatism OU as well as steepening and mild distortion
     of keratometry readings OU. He has a positive Munson sign. The
     clinician should consider additional testing to rule out:
     a. interstitial keratitis
     b. Graves' disease
     c. keratoconus
     d. recurrent corneal erosion

18. Which of the following would be a useful topical agent in the treatment of fungal keratitis?
   a. vidarabine
   b. natamycin
   c. erythromycin
   d. Neomycin/Bacitracin combination
   e. fluoromethalone

19. A Kayser-Fleischer ring is diagnostic and pathognomonic of ocular involvement of which disease?
   a. Stevens-Johnson syndrome
   b. Wilson's disease
   c. Graves' disease
   d. cystinosis
   e. Richner-Hanhart syndrome

20. Which systemic drug is commonly associated with whorl keratopathy?
   a. amiodarone
   b. prednisone
   c. metformin
   d. lisinopril
   e. Plaquenil

21. Arcus senilis is commonly associated with which systemic condition?
   a. coronary artery disease
   b. diabetes mellitus
   c. hyperlipidemia
   d. Crohn's disease
   e. sarcoidosis

22. Topical application of corticosteroids would be indicated in all of the following conditions EXCEPT:
   a. contact dermatitis
   b. atopic dermatitis
   c. psoriasis
   d. rosacea

23. Avellino corneal dystrophy represents a combination of which two corneal dystrophies?
   a. macular and lattice
   b. granular and lattice
   c. ABMD and Meesman's
   d. Meesman's and lattice

24. The term "microcornea" implies a corneal diameter of _____ mm.
    a. <15
    b. <10
    c. <8
    d. <12

25. Reis-Buckler's corneal dystrophy affects which part of the cornea?
    a. Descemet's membrane
    b. Bowman's layer
    c. stroma
    d. endothelium

26. What systemic condition may be associated with lattice corneal dystrophy?
    a. hyperlipidemia
    b. tuberculosis
    c. anemia
    d. amyloidosis
    e. syphilis

27. The apex of the corneal cone in keratoconus is usually found:
    a. in the central cornea
    b. inferonasal
    c. inferotemporal
    d. superotemporal
    e. superonasal

28. Which of the following is NOT a clinical sign of keratoconus?
    a. Fleischer's ring
    b. Vogt's striae
    c. Munson's sign
    d. increased visibility of corneal nerves
    e. guttata

29. Which surgical procedure is indicated for the long-term rehabilitation of advanced keratoconus?
    a. penetrating keratoplasty
    b. photorefractive keratectomy
    c. thermokeratoplasty
    d. radial keratotomy

30. What is the iron line noted on the cornea at the leading edge of an inactive pterygium termed?
    a. Hudson-Stahli line
    b. Ferry's line
    c. Stocker's line
    d. Fleischer's ring

31. A rare bilateral condition in which the entire cornea is uniformly thinned is:
  a. keratoconus
  b. megalocornea
  c. keratoglobus
  d. pellucid marginal dystrophy

32. Band keratopathy is confined to the:
  a. superior cornea
  b. peripheral cornea
  c. interpalpebral fissure area
  d. central cornea

33. Which of the following disorders is most likely to have an early onset (during the preschool years)?
  a. compound nevocellular nevus
  b. atopic dermatitis
  c. psoriasis
  d. rosacea

34. A _____ is defined as a triangular, fibrovascular connective tissue overgrowth of bulbar conjunctiva onto the cornea.
  a. keloid
  b. pinguecula
  c. phlyctenule
  d. pterygium

35. The stroma makes up what percentage of overall corneal thickness in a healthy eye?
  a. 75%
  b. 50%
  c. 90%
  d. 10%
  e. 66%

36. Which clinical test is useful for measuring corneal thickness?
  a. pachymetry
  b. ultrasound A scan
  c. exophthalmometry
  d. potential acuity meter
  e. tonometry

37. Which of the following does NOT play a role in maintaining optimal corneal dehydration?
     a. stromal swelling pressure
     b. endothelial pump
     c. intraocular pressure
     d. uveoscleral outflow

38. The most significant symptom of Thygeson's keratitis is typically what?
     a. significantly blurred vision
     b. photophobia
     c. pain
     d. foreign body sensation

39. A patient develops neurotrophic keratopathy following a bout of herpes zoster ophthalmicus. Which of the following therapies would be the BEST therapeutic option to lessen the severity of the keratopathy once it has already developed?
     a. induced temporary ptosis via botulinum toxin injection
     b. topical corticosteroid therapy
     c. topical antibiotic therapy
     d. oral antiviral therapy

40. Which of the following is MOST likely to be associated with nodular anterior scleritis?
     a. hypertension
     b. rheumatoid arthritis
     c. extended contact lens wear
     d. keratoconus

41. An advancing pterygium is MOST likely to cause:
     a. with-the-rule astigmatism
     b. against-the-rule astigmatism
     c. hyperopia
     d. myopia

42. What type of corneal infection is characterized by ring infiltrates?
     a. Acanthamoeba
     b. *Pseudomonas*
     c. *Staphylococcus*
     d. *Candida albicans*

43. The most common cause of corneal blindness in developed countries is:
     a. *Acanthamoeba* keratitis
     b. keratoconjunctivitis sicca
     c. herpes simplex keratitis
     d. bullous keratopathy

44. Hyperthyroidism would mimic an intraorbital mass in which of the following ways?
    a. exophthalmos
    b. acute onset of diplopia
    c. early onset (premature) of dry eye symptoms
    d. laboratory findings are identical
    e. a and b

45. A phlyctenule is most often associated with _____ but may be related to _____.
    a. staphylococcal infection, sarcoidosis
    b. streptococcal infection, sarcoidosis
    c. staphylococcal infection, tuberculosis
    d. streptococcal infection, tuberculosis

46. Topical corticosteroid therapy is contraindicated in herpetic _____, but useful in herpetic _____.
    a. stromal keratitis, epithelial keratitis
    b. epithelial keratitis, stromal keratitis
    c. stromal keratitis, remission
    d. epithelial keratitis, remission

47. Topical corticosteroids are not useful for long-term treatment of corneal inflammation because:
    a. their effect diminishes with extended use
    b. extended use may lead to cataract formation
    c. they are not effective antiinflammatory agents
    d. they may lead to corneal melt

48. Which type of keratitis is NOT likely to have associated lid lesions?
    a. herpes zoster keratitis
    b. molluscum contagiosum keratitis
    c. chickenpox keratitis
    d. adenoviral keratitis

49. Decreased corneal sensitivity may be associated with which of the following infections?
    a. bacterial corneal ulcer
    b. *Acanthamoeba* keratitis
    c. herpes simplex keratitis
    d. corneal abrasion

50. In the treatment of herpetic keratitis, trifluridine 1% gtts should be administered:
    a. once daily
    b. three times daily
    c. six times daily
    d. nine times daily
    e. hourly

51. The term "herpes zoster ophthalmicus" is applied when:
    a. vesicular lesions appear
    b. the virus infects the ophthalmic branch of the trigeminal nerve
    c. dendritic corneal lesions are present
    d. the patient experiences reduced corneal sensitivity
    e. the virus infects the facial nerve

52. Which of the following would be the most appropriate treatment for a phlyctenule?
    a. Vigamox QID
    b. Zymar QID
    c. Tobramycin QID
    d. Tobradex QID

53. In terms of zoster infection, Hutchinson's sign occurs when:
    a. the zoster infection results in corneal involvement
    b. the cutaneous infection respects the midline
    c. the side of the tip of the nose is involved
    d. the upper lip is involved

54. Hutchinson's sign indicates what nerve is involved in the zoster infection?
    a. nasociliary branch of the trigeminal
    b. frontal branch of the trigeminal
    c. lacrimal branch of the trigeminal
    d. facial nerve

55. Erythematous facial lesions may occur in tumorous as well as inflammatory processes. Which of these disorders will not appear on both sides of the midline?
    a. DLE
    b. Sturge-Weber
    c. psoriasis
    d. seborrheic blepharitis
    e. congenital (hair) nevus

56. What is the significance of Hutchinson's sign to the optometrist?
    a. it indicates the severity of the varicella infection
    b. it can be a predictor of ophthalmic involvement
    c. it always coincides with corneal disease
    d. when present, it means that the infection is subsiding

57. Herpes zoster ophthalmicus can directly result in all of the following EXCEPT:
    a. iridocyclitis
    b. retinitis
    c. extraocular muscle palsy
    d. noninflammatory glaucoma
    e. scleritis

58. A differentiating feature between simplex dendritic lesions and zoster dendritic lesions is:
    a. zoster lesions do not stain with Rose Bengal
    b. corneal sensitivity may be decreased
    c. zoster dendrites do not exhibit end bulbs
    d. zoster does not cause dendritic corneal lesions

59. Herpes zoster keratitis is most effectively managed with:
    a. topical trifluridine
    b. oral acyclovir
    c. topical corticosteroids
    d. oral analgesics

60. Which of the following is a topical antifungal medication?
    a. fluconazole
    b. natamycin
    c. erythromycin
    d. Neomycin

61. Reepithelialization after PRK normally occurs within:
    a. 1 day
    b. 2 to 4 days
    c. 1 week
    d. 1 month

62. All of the following are potential sources of reduced acuity after PRK EXCEPT:
    a. spherical aberration
    b. irregular refraction caused by the transition zone
    c. central islands
    d. "sands of Sahara"

63. Clinical symptoms of central islands include all of the following EXCEPT:
    a. pain
    b. blurred vision
    c. monocular diplopia
    d. glare

64. Staphylococcal hypersensitivity keratitis is characterized by which of the following?
    a. central corneal infiltrates
    b. significantly blurred vision
    c. limbal infiltrates at 3 and 9 o'clock
    d. inferior limbal infiltrates

65. The most important agent in the reduction of corneal haze after PRK is a(an):
    a. topical antibiotic
    b. topical steroid
    c. oral steroid
    d. ocular lubricants

66. Of the following lesions, which one will NOT have pearly raised edges or a dimpled (depressed) center?
    a. keratocanthoma
    b. molluscum contagiosum
    c. basal cell carcinoma
    d. psoriasis

67. Which of the following is an absolute contraindication for refractive surgery?
    a. diabetes mellitus
    b. keratoconus
    c. high astigmatism
    d. chronic dry eye

68. A 12-D myope would be best suited for which refractive surgery technique?
    a. laser-assisted in situ keratomileusis
    b. photorefractive keratectomy
    c. thermokeratoplasty
    d. incisional keratotomy

69. "Sands of Sahara" are:
    a. debris trapped under the corneal flap
    b. central corneal guttata
    c. inflammation in the lamellar interface
    d. folds of the corneal flap

70. Central islands are defined as an area on topography that shows at least _____ of steepening at least _____ in diameter.
   a. 3.00 D, 1.5 mm
   b. 2.50 D, 1.5 mm
   c. 3.50 D, 2.0 mm
   d. 3.00 D, 2.0 mm
   e. 2.50 D, 2.0 mm

71. Which of the following is NOT true for intrastromal corneal ring implants?
   a. glare and night vision problems are significant side effects
   b. the rings are made of PMMA
   c. implantation is irreversible
   d. their insertion channels are made at two-thirds corneal depth

72. Contact lens wearers who use distilled water and salt tablets instead of commercially prepared saline solutions are at increased risk for the development of:
   a. *Acanthamoeba* keratitis
   b. luetic keratitis
   c. superior limbic keratoconjunctivitis
   d. Terrien's marginal keratitis

73. Nummular keratitis is frequently associated with herpes zoster ophthalmicus. In general, it occurs how long after the onset of the skin rash?
   a. 1 days
   b. 3 days
   c. 1 to 2 weeks
   d. >2 weeks

74. Dellen are frequently found in the _____ cornea and are associated with _____.
   a. central, infection
   b. peripheral, contact lens wear
   c. central, dystrophy
   d. peripheral, dystrophy
   e. peripheral, adjacent raised mass

75. Which is the LEAST common sign in epithelial basement membrane dystrophy?
   a. maps
   b. dots
   c. fingerprints
   d. maps and fingerprints in combination
   e. maps and dots in combination

76. The MOST common distribution of SPK associated with staphylococcal toxicity is:
    a. superior
    b. diffuse
    c. inferior
    d. central band

77. Cutaneous nevocellular nevi undergo three stages during their development. Although both congenital nevi and nevocellular nevi are flat in the initial presentation, congenital nevi have the potential to undergo malignant transformation. The characteristic clinical feature of congenital nevi distinguishing them from nevocellular nevi is:
    a. the presence of coarse hair on the congenital nevus
    b. elevation of the congenital nevus
    c. greenish-gray color of the congenital nevus
    d. presence of coarse hair and greenish-gray color of the congenital variety

78. Fungal keratitis must be seriously considered in any case that presents with:
    a. ring infiltrates
    b. phlyctenule
    c. history of contact lens wear
    d. history of vegetative injury
    e. recurrent corneal erosion

79. Seidel's sign (percolation effect) is seen in cases of:
    a. fungal keratitis
    b. corneal perforation
    c. infectious keratitis
    d. herpes simplex keratitis

80. Which of the following is(are) TRUE concerning stromal keratitis associated with herpes simplex infection?
    a. it is rarely seen in primary infection
    b. it may be found with or without the presence of an epithelial dendrite
    c. steroids should not be used in the management of stromal herpetic keratitis
    d. a and b
    e. a, b, and c

81. An eschar is associated with what type of corneal injury?
    a. thermal burn
    b. chemical burn
    c. radiation burn
    d. penetrating injury
    e. corneal abrasion

82. Which of the following is considered to be a TRUE ocular emergency?
    a. thermal corneal burn
    b. chemical corneal burn
    c. fungal corneal infection
    d. *Acanthamoeba* infection
    e. deep corneal abrasion

83. The most important aspect of assessing a corneal foreign body injury is:
    a. removing the foreign body
    b. checking for a secondary anterior chamber reaction
    c. ruling out corneal penetration
    d. initiating pressure patch treatment
    e. removing any associated rust ring

84. Recurrent erosions occur because of damage to:
    a. the stroma
    b. Bowman's layer
    c. the endothelium
    d. Descemet's membrane

85. Arcus senilis occurs at the level of:
    a. the stroma
    b. Bowman's layer
    c. the endothelium
    d. Descemet's membrane

86. Band keratopathy is the result of _____ accumulation in the cornea.
    a. calcium
    b. lipid
    c. inflammatory cells
    d. iron

87. Patients with dendritic herpetic keratitis often experience which of the following symptoms?
    a. photophobia
    b. decreased vision
    c. foreign body sensation
    d. a, b, and c

88. Pigmented tumors are typically rare among Asians or African-Americans. One exception to this general rule is:
    a. malignant melanoma of the palpebral conjunctiva
    b. nevus of Ota
    c. lentigines
    d. keratocanthoma

89. Bullous keratopathy occurs as the result of:
    a. secondary infection
    b. corneal dystrophy
    c. prolonged corneal edema
    d. congenital weakness of the corneal endothelium

90. Bullous keratopathy can result from all of the following EXCEPT:
    a. postoperative complication
    b. corneal degeneration
    c. Fuchs' endothelial dystrophy
    d. herpes zoster ophthalmicus

91. All of the following are treatments for bullous keratopathy EXCEPT:
    a. bandage contact lens
    b. topical antibiotics
    c. penetrating keratoplasty
    d. photorefractive keratectomy

92. A 60-year-old man presents with red, painful eyes. Slit lamp examination reveals groupings of large, peripheral microcysts in each eye with overlying epithelial erosion. Which of the following should be considered in the differential diagnosis?
    a. herpes simplex keratitis
    b. Cogan's microcystic degeneration
    c. Axenfeld's anomaly
    d. keratoconus
    e. Fuchs' endothelial dystrophy

93. Hassal-Henle bodies are:
    a. peripheral guttata
    b. stromal cysts
    c. corneal iron deposits
    d. epithelial microcysts

94. All of the following are true of pterygia EXCEPT they:
    a. result from UV exposure
    b. can be bilateral
    c. tend to progress slowly
    d. are avascular tissue overgrowths

95. Patients with a sterile, hypoxic corneal infiltrate secondary to contact lens wear often have or experience which of the following?
    a. photophobia
    b. anterior chamber reaction
    c. large epithelial defect overlying the infiltrate
    d. a, b, and c

96. Which of the following is NOT a thinning disorder of the cornea?
    a. keratoconus
    b. marginal furrow degeneration
    c. pellucid degeneration
    d. Terrien's marginal degeneration
    e. Salzmann's nodular degeneration

97. Fleischer's ring is a deposition of _____ in the cornea and is associated with _____.
    a. iron, keratoglobus
    b. iron, keratoconus
    c. copper, keratoconus
    d. calcium, keratoglobus
    e. pigment, keratoconus

98. Hudson-Stahli lines occur at the level of:
    a. the epithelium
    b. the stroma
    c. Bowman's layer
    d. Descemet's membrane

99. Basal cell and squamous cell carcinomas will arise from epithelial cells. Important in the clinical differential diagnosis of these malignant entities from keratocanthoma is:
    a. self-resolution of keratocanthoma
    b. self-resolution of BCC/SCC
    c. prevalence for the facial area is high among the malignant varieties
    d. only surgical removal and biopsy will distinguish among these three

100. Krukenberg's spindle is associated with:
    a. keratoconus
    b. pigment dispersion syndrome
    c. ocular albinism
    d. bullous keratopathy

101. Corneal salmon patch is pathognomonic of:
    a. acute corneal hypoxia
    b. syphilitic keratitis
    c. neovascular glaucoma
    d. Sjögren's syndrome

102. Stocker's line is associated with:
    a. pinguecula
    b. pterygia
    c. uveitis
    d. posterior keratoconus

103. Corneal pannus is a frequent complication of which of the following conditions?
    a. histoplasmosis
    b. thyroid disease
    c. rosacea
    d. syphilis

104. Corneal infiltrates are composed of:
    a. iron
    b. fluid
    c. white blood cells
    d. calcium

105. All of the following are treatments for filamentary keratitis EXCEPT:
    a. manual filament removal
    b. bandage contact lens
    c. lubrication
    d. topical steroids

106. Corneal filaments are:
    a. epithelial outgrowths
    b. dead epithelial cells combined with mucin strands
    c. mucin and lipid strands
    d. viral strands adhered to the corneal surface

107. A phlyctenule is a(an):
    a. localized infiltrative reaction
    b. neovascular response
    c. accumulation of red blood cells
    d. pterygium

108. Phlyctenular keratoconjunctivitis can be associated with what systemic disease?
    a. sarcoidosis
    b. syphilis
    c. tuberculosis
    d. coronary artery disease

109. All of the following are true of Thygeson's superficial punctate keratitis EXCEPT:
    a. is often asymptomatic
    b. etiology is unknown
    c. tends to be a self-limiting condition
    d. usually associated with underlying collagen vascular disease

110. Which of the following would NOT be likely among younger patients (under age 40)?
    a. BCC
    b. epidermal inclusion cyst
    c. acrochordon
    d. seborrheic keratosis

111. Which of the following drugs would NOT be appropriate for monotherapy of a sight-threatening corneal ulcer?
    a. tobramycin
    b. Zymar
    c. Vigamox
    d. a, b, and c

112. One of the most common contagious clinical conditions managed in primary eye care is:
    a. bacterial corneal ulcer
    b. herpes simplex keratitis
    c. epidemic keratoconjunctivitis
    d. interstitial keratitis

113. The most common cause of epidemic keratoconjunctivitis (EKC) is:
    a. adenovirus
    b. herpesvirus
    c. *Staphylococcus*
    d. *Staphylococcus aureus*
    e. idiopathic

114. Corneal SPK presentation in epidemic keratoconjunctivitis usually begins approximately:
    a. within 24 hours of infection
    b. on day 3 of infection
    c. on day 8 of infection
    d. 2 weeks or longer after initial exposure

115. In cases of epidemic keratoconjunctivitis, subepithelial infiltrates (SEIs) are expected to appear:
    a. within the first 24 to 48 hours
    b. after 1 week
    c. after 2 weeks
    d. SEIs are not associated with EKC

116. Pharyngoconjunctival fever is found most commonly in:
    a. the elderly
    b. the pediatric population
    c. underdeveloped nations
    d. AIDS patients

117. All of the following are TRUE of pharyngoconjunctival fever
EXCEPT:
a. is an adenoviral infection
b. has systemic manifestations
c. will have associated preauricular lymphadenopathy
d. must be aggressively treated with topical agents

118. Which of the following pharmaceutical agents would NOT routinely
be used to manage a corneal abrasion?
a. cycloplegics
b. antibiotics
c. steroids
d. nonsteroidal antiinflammatory agents

119. The etiology of adult inclusion keratitis is:
a. acne rosacea
b. *Chlamydia*
c. fungus
d. adenovirus
e. autoimmune disease

120. All of the following are TRUE for neonatal inclusion conjunctivitis
EXCEPT:
a. most frequent cause of conjunctivitis in infants
b. risk of transmission from infected mother is greater than 20%
c. frequently associated with a pneumonia-like upper respiratory
infection
d. is a self-limiting condition

121. An effective oral medication for the treatment of neonatal inclusion
conjunctivitis is:
a. tetracycline
b. erythromycin
c. acyclovir
d. Bacitracin

122. Sun exposure is a risk factor in many cutaneous neoplasms. Which of
the following would NOT have ultraviolet radiation as a potentiating
factor?
a. seborrheic keratosis
b. actinic keratosis
c. BCC
d. Bowen's disease (intraepithelial epithelioma)

123. Pellucid marginal degeneration typically affects the:
    a. inferior cornea
    b. superior cornea
    c. central cornea
    d. entire limbal area

124. Terrien's marginal degeneration typically thins the:
    a. inferior cornea
    b. superior cornea
    c. central cornea
    d. entire limbal area

125. All of the following are true of Mooren's ulcer EXCEPT:
    a. usually a limbal presentation
    b. no discharge
    c. frequently has associated neovascularization
    d. usually appears in the first decade of life

Answers

1. a. Corneal ulcers, whether sterile or infectious, always begin with an epithelial defect.

2. b. Chronic hypoxia of the cornea, particularly with extended contact lens wear, leads to corneal epithelial microcysts.

3. c. Sterile infiltrates tend to be more peripheral and less painful and have little anterior chamber reaction compared with infectious ulcers. Corneal scars do not stain.

4. d. Topical steroids slow the healing process and are contraindicated for corneal abrasions.

5. a. Corneal guttata appear in the earliest stages of Fuchs' endothelial dystrophy and are considered a hallmark clinical sign of the condition.

6. d. Corneal guttata are abnormalities of Descemet's membrane.

7. d. Granular is a stromal dystrophy.

8. c. MDF dystrophy is an epithelial basement membrane dystrophy of the cornea.

9. a. Corneal dystrophies usually are hereditary, bilateral, and progressive and are not associated with systemic or local disease.

10. c. Dots are intraepithelial microcysts that contain nuclear, cytoplasmic, and lipid debris.

11. a. While psoriasis affects many people worldwide, contact dermatitis remains the leading cause of eyelid eruption.

12. c. The most common clinical presentation of herpes simplex keratitis is a dendritic corneal ulcer.

13. d. Topical steroids are contraindicated in the initial treatment of herpes simplex keratitis because they exacerbate the disease. They may be used several days later to quell the immune response in the presence of stromal disease.

14. a. Syphilis is the leading cause of interstitial keratitis.

15. a. PPD is an endothelial dystrophy.

16. b. Inadequate tear film protection leads to desiccation of the cornea and keratoconjunctivitis sicca.

17. c. Early signs of keratoconus include increase in myopia and astigmatism, steepening of keratometry readings, distortion of keratometry mires and a positive Munson's sign (V-shaped pattern to lower lid on downgaze).

18. b. Natamycin is a topical antifungal agent.

19. b. A Kayser-Fleischer ring is a copper deposit ring that is diagnostic of Wilson's disease.

20. a. Whorl keratopathy is a side effect of amiodarone therapy.

21. c. Arcus senilis is the deposition of cholesterol in the corneal tissue commonly found in patients with hyperlipidemia.

22. d. Each of the distracters is an inflammatory condition that is localized. Rosacea is thought to have a bacterial systemic etiology with ocular manifestations *(Helicobacter pylori)*.

23. b. Avellino is a combination of granular and lattice dystrophies.

24. b. The term microcornea implies a corneal diameter of less than 10 mm.

25. b. Reis-Buckler's corneal dystrophy is a superficial dystrophy of Bowman's layer.

26. d. Lattice degeneration is commonly seen in patients with systemic amyloidosis.

27. b. The apex of the corneal cone in keratoconus is usually displaced inferonasally.

28. e. Guttata are not typically associated with keratoconus.

29. a. Penetrating keratoplasty (corneal transplant surgery) is indicated for the long-term treatment of advanced keratoconus.

30. c. Stocker's line forms as the result of long-time tear pooling at the edge of an inactive pterygium.

31. c. Keratoglobus is a rare bilateral condition in which the cornea is uniformly thinned, particularly peripherally.

32. c. Band keratopathy is restricted to the interpalpebral fissure area.

33. b. Only atopic dermatitis is not an acquired disorder.

34. d. A pterygium is defined as a triangular, fibrovascular connective tissue overgrowth of bulbar conjunctiva onto the cornea.

35. c. The stroma accounts for 90% of normal corneal thickness.

36. a. Pachymetry is a useful tool for measuring corneal thickness.

37. d. Preservation of adequate corneal dehydration results from the following five factors: stromal swelling pressure (SP), the barrier function of the epithelium and endothelium, the endothelial pump, evaporation from the corneal surface, and the intraocular pressure (IOP).

38. b. The entering complaint of patients with Thygeson's keratitis is usually photophobia. Blurring of vision is usually mild, and there is little pain or foreign body sensation.

39. a. Neurotrophic keratopathy may occur when there is disrupted innervation to the cornea. The best treatment measure is to prevent corneal desiccation. Frequent instillation of artificial tears is often inadequate, and the cornea may best be protected by eyelid coverage. Topical corticosteroids, antibiotics, and antivirals will not improve the innervational deficit to the cornea.

40. b. Scleritis is most likely to be associated with concurrent collagen vascular disease. Hypertension, contact lens wear, and keratoconus have no known association with scleritis.

41. a. As a pterygium advances, it is most likely to cause flattening of the 180-degree corneal meridian and progressive with-the-rule astigmatism.

42. a. *Acanthamoeba* infection is characterized by ring infiltrates once stromal infection has occurred.

43. c. Herpes simplex infection is the most common cause of corneal blindness in developed countries.

44.   a.   Diplopia may be related to restriction of global movement, but acute diplopia is typically neurologic. In hyperthyroidism, there is infiltration of the extraocular muscles that causes exophthalmos via a different mechanism than intraorbital mass.

45.   c.   Phlyctenules are most commonly seen with staphylococcal infection but may be related to tuberculosis proteins or antibodies.

46.   b.   Topical corticosteroid therapy is contraindicated in herpetic epithelial keratitis because it exacerbates the disease. Topical corticosteroids are useful in herpetic stromal keratitis for their ability to control underlying inflammation.

47.   b.   Extended use of topical corticosteroids may lead to formation of posterior subcapsular cataract.

48.   d.   Adenoviral infections are not expected to have associated lid lesions.

49.   c.   Decreased corneal sensitivity can occur with herpes simplex keratitis, particularly in recurrent herpetic corneal disease.

50.   d.   Topical trifluridine 1% is typically administered nine times per day for the treatment of herpes simplex keratitis.

51.   b.   The term herpes zoster ophthalmicus applies when the ophthalmic branch of the trigeminal nerve is involved.

52.   d.   Tobradex would be the most appropriate agent from this list because it combines an antibiotic and a steroid.

53.   c.   Hutchinson's sign is positive when the side of the tip of the nose (not just the tip) is involved.

54.   a.   Hutchinson's sign is an indicator that the nasociliary branch of the trigeminal nerve has been infected.

55.   b.   Although one case has been reported in the literature, unilaterality is the hallmark of Sturge-Weber syndrome.

56.   b.   Hutchinson's sign can be an indicator of ophthalmic involvement.

57.   d.   HZO can cause blepharitis, canaliculitis, conjunctivitis, dacryoadenitis, keratitis, keratouveitis, iridocyclitis, vitritis, retinitis, acute retinal necrosis, retinal vasculitis, choroiditis, inflammatory glaucoma, optic neuritis, meningeal encephalitis, inflammatory extraocular muscle palsies, anterior segment ischemia, episcleritis, scleritis, postherpetic neuralgia, and cephalalgia.

58. c. Zoster dendrites do not exhibit terminal end-bulb formation.

59. b. Zoster ophthalmicus is most effectively managed with oral acyclovir. Topical antivirals have little effect.

60. b. Natamycin is available as a topical antifungal agent. Fluconazole is an oral antifungal.

61. b. Complete reepithelialization after PRK normally occurs within 2 to 4 days.

62. d. Sands of Sahara is a LASIK complication.

63. a. Pain is not a typical symptom of central island formation. Central islands cause visual side effects.

64. d. Inferior limbal infiltrates are observed because this is where the lid margin is in contact with the cornea–limbus. Superior infiltrates are also possible at the lid–cornea junction but are not as common.

65. b. Topical steroids are usually used in the reduction of postoperative corneal haze in PRK patients.

66. d. Keratocanthoma and BCC both have pearly edges and dimpled centers. Molluscum, while of viral etiology, may have the same appearance.

67. b. Keratoconus is an absolute contraindication due to preexisting corneal thinning.

68. a. LASIK is usually the best procedure for correction of high myopia.

69. c. Sands of Sahara represent a nonspecific inflammation in the lamellar interface.

70. a. Central islands are defined as an area on topography that shows, at minimum, 3.00 D of steepening at least 1.5 mm in diameter.

71. c. Intacs can be removed (explanted) if complications arise.

72. a. Luetic keratitis refers to keratitis associated with syphilis. Terrien's marginal keratitis and superior limbic keratoconjunctivitis are noninfectious and have no association with distilled water and salt tablet use. Contact lens wearers can develop a contact lens-associated SLK, but this has no known relationship to distilled water and salt tablet use.

73. c. On average, nummular keratitis occurs about 10 days after the onset of the skin rash associated with herpes zoster ophthalmicus.

74. e. Dellen are found in the peripheral cornea and are frequently associated with an adjacent raised mass.

75. c. Fingerprints are the least common clinical sign in MDF dystrophy.

76. c. SPK associated with staphylococcal toxicity is most commonly found on the inferior cornea.

77. a. Coarse hair is a consistent feature of congenital nevi that has been identified as a clinical feature consistent with malignant potential (although low).

78. d. A history of vegetative injury, such as a tree branch abrasion, must make the clinician wary of secondary fungal infection.

79. b. Seidel's sign is an indicator of corneal penetration or perforation.

80. d. Steroids are often needed to combat stromal inflammation and scarring in herpetic keratitis involving the stroma. Topical antivirals (Viroptic) are typically used in conjunction with the steroid to minimize the likelihood of dendrite formation. Stromal disease is almost never observed with primary infection, only recurrent secondary outbreaks.

81. a. An eschar is a mass of whitish-gray "charred" epithelial cells associated with thermal burns of the cornea.

82. b. A chemical corneal burn is considered to be a true ocular emergency requiring immediate intervention in order to save vision.

83. c. Corneal penetration must be ruled out in all cases of corneal foreign body injury.

84. b. RCE is a result of damage or weakness in Bowman's layer of the cornea.

85. b. Arcus senilis occurs at the level of Bowman's layer.

86. a. Band keratopathy results from the accumulation of calcium in the cornea.

87. d. All of these symptoms occur with dendritic herpes simplex keratitis (HSK).

88. b. As the name suggests, the initial report was from Japan.

89. c. Bullous keratopathy occurs as the result of prolonged corneal edema.

90. d. Bullous keratopathy is not an outcome of herpes zoster ophthalmicus.

91. d. PRK is a refractive surgery technique and not indicated for bullous keratopathy.

92. b. Cogan's microcystic degeneration is classified as unilateral or bilateral groupings of large epithelial microcysts, sometimes with painful erosion.

93. a. Hassal-Henle bodies (also called Descemet's warts) are peripheral corneal guttata.

94. d. Pterygia are richly vascularized.

95. a. A significant epithelial defect overlying a stromal infiltrate is a corneal ulcer, not a sterile infiltrate, and anterior chamber reactions are more often associated with corneal ulcers than sterile infiltrates. Photophobia is very common with sterile hypoxic keratitis.

96. e. Salzmann's nodular degeneration manifests as formations of elevated gray-blue nodules on the corneal surface. There is no associated corneal thinning.

97. b. Fleischer's ring is a deposition of iron in the cornea and is associated with keratoconus.

98. c. Hudson-Stahli lines occur at the level of Bowman's layer in the band region (interpalpebral region) of the cornea.

99. a. Keratocanthoma will typically self-resolve due to its rapid growth within about 6 months. Longer-standing lesions should have biopsy for definitive diagnosis.

100. b. Krukenberg's spindle is usually associated with either pigment dispersion syndrome or old uveitis.

101. b. Salmon patch is a finding associated with interstitial keratitis and is pathognomonic of syphilitic keratitis.

102. a. Stocker's line is a line of ferrous deposits found at the leading edge of pterygia.

103. c. Pannus is frequently observed in rosacea patients.

104. c. Corneal infiltrates are accumulations of white blood cells in the cornea.

105. d. Unless indicated in the treatment of an underlying disease, topical steroids are not a typical treatment for filamentary keratitis.

106. b. Corneal filaments are dead epithelial cells combined with mucin and adhered to dry patches on the corneal surface.

107. a. A phlyctenule is a localized infiltrative superficial reaction on the cornea.

108. c. Phlyctenular keratoconjunctivitis is associated with tuberculosis, particularly in underdeveloped countries.

109. d. There are no systemic associations with Thygeson's SPK. The etiology is unknown.

110. a. BCC is the most common periocular tumor, and incidence increases with age. The others are common among all age groups.

111. a. Fourth-generation fluoroquinolones (Vigamox and Zymar) are acceptable for monotherapy of bacterial corneal ulcers, but tobramycin is not. It can be used, but not as stand-alone therapy.

112. c. EKC is a common and highly contagious viral keratoconjunctivitis.

113. a. EKC is an adenoviral infection.

114. c. According to the "rule of 8s," corneal SPK findings generally present on approximately the eighth day of infection.

115. c. SEIs generally appear after 2 weeks or more of EKC infection.

116. b. PCF is an adenoviral infection affecting primarily small children.

117. d. PCF is a viral infection and must be allowed to "run its course" with possible lubricant or decongestant therapy for symptoms as needed.

118. c. Steroids are not typically part of corneal abrasion therapy, while all of the other agents are.

119. b. Adult inclusion keratitis is a result of chlamydial infection.

120. d. Neonatal inclusion conjunctivitis must be aggressively treated to prevent pannus and corneal scarring.

121. b. Oral erythromycin is an effective treatment for inclusion conjunctivitis in neonates. Bacitracin does not come in oral forms.

122. a. Actinic, as the name implies, is related to sun exposure; BCC is also. Seborrheic keratosis occurs more frequently in African-American patients and is not related to sun exposure.

123. a. Pellucid marginal degeneration typically affects the inferior cornea.

124. b. Terrien's marginal degeneration typically thins the superior cornea.

125. d. Mooren's ulcer generally appears in the older patient population.

Glaucoma

Leo P. Semes

1. Which of the following sequences represents the contemporary progression from normal to blindness (the ultimate outcome of glaucoma)?
    a. normal, GCL loss, NFL loss, vascular changes, VF damage
    b. normal, vascular changes, NFL loss, VF damage
    c. normal, GCL loss, NFL loss, VF damage
    d. neither; each patient is different

2. Which of the following is a component of the contemporary definition of glaucoma?
    a. progressive optic neuropathy
    b. progressive visual field changes
    c. elevated IOP
    d. only a and b are components of the contemporary definition of glaucoma
    e. a, b, and c

3. Which of the following is the most significant risk factor for developing glaucoma?
    a. ONH cupping
    b. visual field defect
    c. progression
    d. elevated IOP

4. Which of the following is not a component of the glaucoma risk calculator (GRC)?
    a. age
    b. race
    c. IOP
    d. CCT
    e. PSD

5.   Which of the following is the BEST definition of target pressure?
  a.   that IOP at which the patient ceases to show progression of the VF or ONH
  b.   that IOP that is at least 30% less than the highest baseline IOP
  c.   that IOP that is more than 20% below the initial IOP
  d.   that IOP that is consistent with reduction expected from the agents used to lower IOP
  e.   that IOP that is the same in each eye and does not fluctuate more than 2 mm Hg throughout a diurnal measurement period

6.   Approximately how many nerve fibers would you expect a normal adult to have?
  a.   500,000
  b.   1,000,000
  c.   1,500,000
  d.   2,000,000
  e.   3,000,000

7.   You measure a patient's IOP to be 28 mm Hg. You then measure a central corneal thickness of 600 μm. What can you definitively say about this patient's true IOP?
  a.   it is 28
  b.   it is 31
  c.   it is 25
  d.   it is higher than 28
  e.   it is lower than 28

8.   Which of the following is NOT a clinical feature of NTG?
  a.   IOP > 24
  b.   localized optic nerve damage
  c.   disc hemorrhage is more common than in POAG
  d.   field loss closer to fixation and steeper

9.   Establishing target pressure for the medical reduction of IOP is important in which of the following diagnostic categories?
  a.   POAG
  b.   NTG
  c.   narrow angle glaucoma
  d.   a and b

10. Your patient is a 68-year-old African-American woman with a history of heart disease who is currently treated for high blood pressure. She has not achieved her "target pressure" with Xalatan, although the drug has reduced IOP about 25%. Which of the following regimens is most likely the best addition?
   a. Betimol alone
   b. timolol plus Alphagan P
   c. Trusopt alone
   d. Cosopt plus Travatan
   e. Alphagan

11. Which of the following can be considered "first-line" treatment of POAG?
   a. beta-blockers
   b. prostaglandin analogs
   c. topical CAIs
   d. alpha$_2$-agonists
   e. a through d could be used first line, depending on patient characteristics

12. For previously untreated patients with POAG, what should be the follow-up interval for the first visit after pharmacotherapy has been initiated?
   a. 3 to 5 days
   b. 1 to 2 weeks
   c. 2 to 4 weeks
   d. 1 to 3 months
   e. >3 months

13. Regarding the CNTGT, which of the following statements is TRUE?
   a. reducing IOP by 30% with medication reduced VF progression at 5 years to 20% (versus 60% in the untreated control group)
   b. reducing IOP by 30% and accounting for cataract, VF progression at 5 years was reduced from 60% to 20%
   c. reducing IOP in patients with normal IOP but high risk of glaucomatous damage was unsuccessful in reducing VF progression
   d. neither a, b, nor c

14. In the CNTGT, which of the following means could be used to lower IOP?
   a. medication
   b. filtering surgery
   c. laser surgery
   d. a, b, or c
   e. neither a, b, nor c; patients were simply observed for progression for 5 years

15. A major outcome of CIGITS was which of the following?
    a. both surgery and medication to lower IOP are successful in slowing progression
    b. surgery was more successful in slowing progression than medication
    c. medication was more successful in slowing progression than surgery
    d. neither surgery nor medication was successful in slowing progression once visual field damage was established

16. From the results of OHTS, which of the following features is NOT significant in the multivariate analysis for predicting conversion from OHT to POAG?
    a. CCT (<555 μm)
    b. higher age
    c. black race
    d. vertical C/D ratio
    e. global index of PSD

17. In OHTS, lowering IOP in those with ocular hypertension reduced the risk of converting to POAG by about how much?
    a. 10%
    b. 20%
    c. 30%
    d. 40%
    e. 50%

18. According to the "rule of fives" from OHTS, which of the following would constitute high risk?
    a. C/D >0.5, CCT >555, IOP >24.75
    b. C/D >0.5, CCT<555, IOP >25.75
    c. age >50, CCT >555, C/D >0.5
    d. age >50, CCT <555, IOP >50
    e. age <50, CCT <555, C/D >0.5

19. In OHTS, conversion from OHT to POAG occurred most frequently from which of the following clinical findings?
    a. disc change
    b. VF change
    c. a and b
    d. elevated IOP at the first three visits

20. In OHTS, investigators could choose any topical medication to lower IOP. Which two medications were prescribed most prevalently?
    a. beta-blockers and prostaglandins
    b. prostaglandins and CAIs
    c. beta-blockers and CAIs
    d. alpha-blockers and beta-blockers

21. Which of the following statements concerning OHTS results is TRUE?
    a. all patients with IOP >24 deserve treatment to prevent conversion to glaucoma
    b. diurnal control is critical to prevent conversion from OHT to glaucoma
    c. CCT was identified as a "powerful risk factor" in predicting who would convert from OHT to glaucoma
    d. none of the medicated patients (IOP ≤ 24% or IOP >20% from baseline) converted
    e. only patients with thin corneas (<555 μm) are at risk to convert to glaucoma

22. Your patient has the following clinical findings: age 56, IOP 23/32 [OD/OS], C/D 0.3/0.6 [OD/OS], reliable and clear visual field, negative family history of glaucoma and open angles. What is(are) the possible diagnosis(es)?
    a. glaucoma suspect
    b. ocular hypertension
    c. POAG
    d. a, b, or c
    e. NTG

23. The class of IOP-lowering medications that provides for most consistent diurnal control with daily administration is the:
    a. beta-blockers
    b. prostaglandins
    c. alpha-agonists
    d. CA inhibitors
    e. alpha-antagonists

24. Which of the following is most likely to remain unchanged if the patient has progressive cataract but stable glaucoma?
    a. MD
    b. PSD
    c. CPSD
    d. SF
    e. LS

25. Which of the following global indices is(are) part of the algorithm that supports the diagnosis of glaucoma?
    a. MD
    b. PSD
    c. CPSD
    d. SF
    e. b or c, depending on strategy

26. Which of the following global indices represents the average of depressions found throughout the visual field?
    a. MD
    b. PSD
    c. CPSD
    d. SF
    e. b or c, depending on strategy

27. Frequency doubling technology (FDT) uses low spatial and high temporal frequency sinusoidal grating as a stimulus target. This combination is thought to be advantageous in the early detection of visual field loss in glaucoma due to which of the following?
    a. M-cell pathways are damaged early in the glaucomatous process
    b. this technology targets the M-cell pathways
    c. the large receptive fields of the LGN are sensitive to these stimuli
    d. a and b

28. Which of the following conditions is NOT an example of 2-degree open-angle glaucoma?
    a. exfoliation
    b. neovascular
    c. posttraumatic
    d. ciliary block
    e. pigmentary

29. Which of the following forms of glaucoma is NOT characterized by pupillary block?
    a. miotic-induced
    b. lens-induced
    c. spherophakia
    d. neovascular

30. Older, hyperopic individuals with small globes and significantly narrow anterior chamber angles are prone to have what type of glaucoma?
    a. pigmentary
    b. angle-closure
    c. exfoliation
    d. neovascular
    e. NTG

31. When managing AACG, which should be avoided if the IOP >40 mm Hg?
    a. topical apraclonidine
    b. topical pilocarpine
    c. topical beta-blockers
    d. oral acetazolamide
    e. topical prostaglandin analogues

32. In the treatment of acute pupillary block AC glaucoma, "definitive" management entails:
    a. laser iridotomy
    b. topical miotics
    c. topical beta-blockers
    d. trabeculectomy
    e. viscocanulostomy

33. The pigment in pigmentary glaucoma is derived from:
    a. the RPE
    b. iris epithelium
    c. ciliary body
    d. endogenous conversion of catecholamines
    e. iris stromal melanocytes

34. Approximately what percentage of patients with PDS can be expected to develop PG?
    a. 10%
    b. 25%
    c. 50%
    d. 75%
    e. 100%

35. The "classic" profile for a patient who develops pigmentary glaucoma is:
    a. hyperopic female in her 20s to 30s
    b. myopic male in his 20s to 30s
    c. hyperopic male in his 50s
    d. male or female with cataract in his or her 70s

36. Which of the following characteristics is not part of the clinical profile of Posner-Schlossman syndrome?
    a. bilateral involvement
    b. age of 20 to 50 years
    c. history of recurrent attacks of blurred vision
    d. open anterior chamber angles without posterior or anterior synechia

37. You decide to dilate a patient with the usual cocktail of tropicamide and phenylephrine. One hour following dilation, you measure IOP and find that it is up 10 mm Hg to 32 mm Hg. On gonioscopy, you confirm that you have caused angle closure. Which of the following medications would be contraindicated in managing the attack?
    a. 4% pilocarpine
    b. oral glycerin
    c. dapiprazole
    d. topical beta-blocker
    e. any of these would be appropriate in the management of AAC attack

38. Which of the following would you NOT find to be consistent with acute angle closure?
    a. swollen optic nerve
    b. mid-dilated pupil, poorly reactive to light
    c. steamy cornea
    d. glaucomflecken
    e. posterior synechiae

39. Which of the following would NOT be an etiology of pupillary block glaucoma?
    a. posterior synechiae from uveitis or trauma
    b. iris bombe
    c. pseudophakia with posterior synechiae
    d. ciliary body rotation
    e. inflammation leading to PAS

40. In retinal vein occlusion, which of the following is the BEST predictor for developing NVG?
    a. presenting VA (>20/200)
    b. CWS
    c. ischemic territory
    d. number and extent of hemorrhages and exudates
    e. IOP at initial observation

41. Management of NVG may include all of the following EXCEPT:
    a. PRP
    b. topical prostaglandins
    c. topical beta-blockers and CAIs
    d. systemic CAIs

42. Which of the following is NOT a component of the ICE syndrome?
    a. Chandler's syndrome (essential iris atrophy)
    b. iris nevus (or Cogan-Reese) syndrome
    c. progressive (essential) iris atrophy
    d. Fuch's heterochromic iridocyclitis
    e. angle recession

43. Your 32-year-old white female patient has a mildly irregular pupil, anterior-chamber abnormalities, and IOP of 36 mm Hg. Which of the following would NOT be a diagnostic candidate?
    a. Axenfeld-Rieger syndrome
    b. ICE syndrome
    c. Peter's anomaly
    d. Fuch's heterochromic iridocyclitis
    e. angle recession

44. Which of the following is a form of open-angle glaucoma?
     a. pigment dispersion
     b. Axenfeld-Rieger syndrome
     c. exfoliation
     d. a and c

45. Your osteoarthritic patient who is taking indomethacin (Indocin, an
     NSAID) presents with the third episode of uveitis and elevated IOP in
     the last 18 months. Which of the following treatment schemes would
     be INAPPROPRIATE?
     a. Pred Forte QID × 1 Wk & RTC
     b. 5% homatropine BID
     c. topical beta-blockers and CAIs
     d. any of the prostaglandins

46. Which of the following would NOT be part of the spectrum of pigment
     dispersion (PD)?
     a. Krukenberg's spindle
     b. iris transillumination
     c. pigment deposition on iris, lens, trabecular meshwork
     d. posterior iris bowing (gonioscopically)
     e. none; all of these *are* part of the spectrum of PD

47. Which of the following would NOT be part of the clinical picture of
     pigment dispersion?
     a. usually diagnosed in the 20s or 30s
     b. 10% to 15% of PDS patients develop PDG
     c. a form of open-angle glaucoma
     d. may be exacerbated by exercise and pupil dilation
     e. none; all of these *are* part of the spectrum of PD

48. Management of glaucoma secondary to pigment dispersion may
     include all of the following EXCEPT:
     a. prostaglandins
     b. pilopine gel
     c. LPI
     d. topical beta-blockers and CAIs

49. Which of the following ocular tissues is typically spared from
     exfoliative deposition?
     a. lens
     b. iris
     c. zonule
     d. TM
     e. none of these are spared

50. Management of exfoliation glaucoma includes all of the following EXCEPT:
    a. typical topicals
    b. ALT
    c. trabeculectomy
    d. LPI

Answers

1. c. Ganglion cell death is the starting point for glaucomatous damage that finally manifests itself as optic disc cupping evident on fundus evaluation and manifested functionally as visual field loss.

2. d. While pressure is the number one risk factor for glaucomatous damage, progressive optic nerve damage is the keystone clinical feature.

3. d. Elevated IOP remains the most significant risk factor and is the only clinical finding for which the FDA approves medication that is used in the treatment of glaucoma.

4. b. Mansberger, in August 2004, extrapolated the risk calculation from results of the OHTS. It includes elements of structure and function but not race as a risk factor. (Mansberger SL: A risk calculator to determine the probability of glaucoma, *Journal of Glaucoma,* 13(4):345-347, 2004.)

5. a. Target IOP is an elusive value, and while there is guidance from large clinical trials as well as the pharmacologic potential of IOP reduction from medications, target IOP is a level at which progression is halted.

6. d. Each optic nerve has about 1 million nerve fibers. A normal adult with two eyes will have 2 million.

7. e. While there are conversion tables based solely on CCT, it is known that factors other than CCT influence the corrected IOP. These may include radius of curvature, for example. The only outcome that can be predicted from a greater-than-average CCT (Goldmann's tonometer is based on 520 CCT) is that the IOP is underestimated.

8. a. The upper limit of IOP is generally accepted as 22 based on 2 standard deviations from the mean of 16.5. NTG would not be consistent with IOP greater than 24.

9. d. The CNTGT and other studies of open-angle glaucoma demonstrate that reducing IOP slows progression. Narrow-angle glaucoma responds best to surgical intervention with peripheral laser iridotomy.

10. c. O'Connor and colleagues showed that dorzolamide twice or three times daily was more effective than brimonidine or beta-blockers when added to latanoprost. (O'Connor DJ, Hsieh JK, Yap D: Additive intraocular pressure lowering effect of various medications with latanoprost, *Am J Ophthalmol* 133:836-937, 2002.)

11. e. All of the beta-blockers and latanaprost have been approved by the FDA for first-line topical treatment of IOP reduction. By extension, the other prostaglandin analogs are included. Additionally, evidence in the literature supports topical CAIs and alpha-agonists.

12. c. Prostaglandin analogs may take up to 3 weeks to show a clinical response. Other medications will do so in a shorter time period.

13. b. This question is from the results of the Collaborative Normal Tension Glaucoma Trial (CNTGT), which demonstrated a treatment benefit for reducing IOP even in normal-tension patients.

14. d. Investigators used both surgery and topical medications to lower IOP. In the end, they discovered that both treatments worked equally well.

15. a. Similar to the results of the CNTGT, both surgery and medication lowered IOP over the course of the study.

16. c. Only African-American race among the elements listed was among the significant risk factors when looking at the elements combined. African-American race was significant in the univariate analysis only.

17. e. This was the classic outcome of the OHTS, which the treatment group converted at 4.4% while the observation group converted at 9.5%.

18. b. Another classic outcome from OHTS was that thinner CCT, larger C/D, and higher IOP were very significant risk factors for conversion from OHT to glaucoma.

19. a. Still another classic finding from the OHTS—55% of conversions were on the basis of disc change, whereas only 35% were on the basis of VF progression and only 10% of patients progressed on both counts.

20. a. At the initiation of OHTS, beta-blockers were used in almost all patients. With the approval of latanaprost, this group of medications gained in use and eventually finished second.

21. c. The OHTS demonstrated that the thinner central cornea was most strongly correlated with conversion. While it is tempting to think that lowering IOP in the treatment group was protective, the threshold mentioned in choice D may have been too high to prevent all conversions.

22. d. In the absence of VF changes correlated with structural damage, this patient could have glaucoma or simply be a suspect of ocular hypertension (elevated IOP in the absence of disc and field changes).

23. b. Several studies have shown that latanaprost is superior to the beta-blockers. Alpha-agonists and CAIs, because of dosing frequency, are unable to reliably keep IOP lowered throughout the diurnal cycle.

24. b. PSD has been shown to remain stationary in the evolution or removal of cataract, for example. Progressive escalation of PSD is evidence of progression of functional damage.

25. e. The Hodapp, Anderson, and Parrish algorithm identifies GHT (outside normal limits), PSD or CPSD flagged and repeated, and clusters as consistent with a diagnosis of glaucoma. (Hodapp E, Parrish RK, Anderson SR: *Clinical decisions in glaucoma,* St Louis, 1993, Mosby.)

26. a. This is a well-known standard.

27. d. This technology does target the M-cell pathways.

28. d. Anatomically, the angle is open in exfoliation, NV, pigmentary, and angle-recession glaucoma.

29. d. Neovascular glaucoma occurs secondary to ischemia. The anterior chamber is open but overgrown with new vessels.

30. b. This is the classic profile of angle closure.

31. b. Pilocarpine will not work when the iris vasculature and neural connections have been rendered ischemic by the elevated IOP greater than 40.

32. a. Among these choices, laser iridotomy is the treatment that will allow aqueous from the posterior to the anterior chambers in phakic individuals.

33. b. Anatomic considerations. The posterior leaf of the iris is the epithelium and pigmented. The peripheral area rubs against the zonules, which liberate melanin granules that show up on the posterior cornea and trabecular meshwork.

34. a. This is the widely cited statistic that was confirmed recently.

35. b. Again, statistically, the most likely people susceptible to PDG are young males.

36. a. All three distracters are true, but the condition is usually unilateral.

37. a. Mapstone showed in the 1970s that all patients with a history of previous attack who were dilated with the adrenergic phenylephrine and underwent attempts to reversal with pilocarpine had papillary block. (Mapstone R: The syndrome of closed-angle glaucoma, *Br J Ophthalmol,* 60:120-123, 1976.)

38. e. As the name suggests, these attacks have rapid onset once the right conditions are present and evolve rapidly.

39. e. Inflammation would be consistent with chronic conditions leading to elevated IOP and chronic angle closure.

40. a. The CVOS showed that this simple finding was predictive of the future devastating consequence during the first 3 postevent years.

41. b. Because prostaglandins may play a role in inflammation, they are contraindicated in the management of NVG.

42. d. Each of the first three represents congenital angle abnormalities; Fuch's is a recurrent inflammatory condition.

43. d. In all but the correct answer, there would be angle abnormalities and the significantly elevated IOP as in the scenario.

44. d. Only A-R will have normal angle.

45. d. Since Indocin is an NSAID, the antagonistic action would rule out prostaglandin use.

46. e. This is a roundabout way of describing the characteristics of PD (items a through d).

47. e. This is another series of descriptors of PD.

48. a. As with NVG, the inflammatory potential of the prostaglandins rules them out in PDG.

49. e. It has been shown that all ocular as well as some systemic tissues are involved in exfoliation.

50. d. As the angle is open, creating an additional orifice would be superfluous.

CHAPTER 22

Lens/Cataract

John B. Crane, Brad M. Sutton, Jennifer A. Palombi

1. A congenital cataract in an infant may cause all of the following EXCEPT:
   a. nystagmus
   b. strabismus
   c. afferent pupillary defect
   d. blunted red reflex

2. Which of the following systemic conditions can lead to refractive error shifts by inducing changes in the refractive index of the lens?
   a. thyroid disease
   b. diabetes
   c. hypertension
   d. lupus erythematosus

3. Which of the following types of cataract usually causes the least visual disability?
   a. nuclear sclerotic
   b. cortical
   c. anterior subcapsular
   d. posterior subcapsular

4. Anterior subcapsular cataracts are often caused by which of the following classes of medication?
   a. steroids
   b. antimalarial agents
   c. phenothiazines
   d. analgesics

5. Which of the following is not a potential expected complication of lens subluxation?
   a. monocular diplopia
   b. pupillary block glaucoma
   c. cataract
   d. angle recession

6. A 72-year-old woman with otherwise healthy eyes has a cataract and a 1.50 D myopic shift in her refraction. What type of cataract does she most likely have?
    a. posterior subcapsular
    b. cortical
    c. congenital
    d. nuclear sclerosis

7. Steroid use can be associated with what kind of cataract?
    a. posterior subcapsular cataract
    b. anterior subcapsular cataract
    c. nuclear sclerotic
    d. cortical

8. A patient presents for cataract evaluation. Which of the following biomicroscopy techniques is least suited for this type of examination?
    a. retroillumination
    b. specular reflection
    c. parallelopiped
    d. slit beam

9. Diabetic patients acquire what type of cataract much more frequently than does the population at large?
    a. nuclear sclerotic
    b. anterior subcapsular
    c. cortical
    d. congenital

10. A patient exhibits phacodonesis in one eye. Which of the following is the LEAST appropriate consideration for the diagnostic etiology?
    a. high myopia
    b. hypermature cataract
    c. ocular trauma
    d. homocystinuria

11. A 30-year-old woman is on chronic high-dose oral prednisone for the treatment of Crohn's disease. What type of cataract is she at risk for developing?
    a. posterior subcapsular
    b. cortical
    c. congenital
    d. nuclear sclerosis

12. Uveitis caused by a hypermature cataract with secondary leakage of lens protein is known as what?
    a. granulomatous uveitis
    b. phacolytic uveitis
    c. phacomorphic uveitis
    d. acute uveitis

13. Which of the following is the LEAST important clinical finding to rule out in your preoperative cataract evaluation?
    a. stromal edema
    b. blepharitis
    c. filtering bleb
    d. punctate epitheliopathy

14. Cataract surgery is most likely to lower intraocular pressure in a patient with which of the following conditions?
    a. high myope
    b. moderate myope
    c. emmetrope
    d. moderate hyperope

15. Which is the following is the BEST reason that keratometry is necessary before a successful cataract surgery outcome can be achieved?
    a. a clear, uniform optical surface of the cornea must be verified
    b. large amounts of corneal astigmatism must be ruled out
    c. refractive power of the cornea is vital to IOL power calculation
    d. keratoconus should be ruled out before surgery is performed

16. Subluxation of the lens may be associated with which of the following systemic disorders?
    a. Marfan's syndrome
    b. diabetes mellitis
    c. temporal arteritis
    d. hyperlipidemia
    e. sarcoidosis

17. Patients with moderate posterior subcapsular cataracts (PSCs) tend to have the most problems with which of the following tasks?
    a. reading
    b. seeing at the beach without sunglasses
    c. driving at night
    d. a and b

18. Which of the following is MOST correct regarding posterior capsular opacification following extracapsular cataract extraction?
    a. thought to be triggered by iris pigment left behind on the capsule
    b. frequency is age related; occurs less often with age
    c. polishing the posterior capsule prevents occurrence
    d. if visual acuity is reduced significantly, an argon laser is used in treatment

Answers

1. c. A cataract alone does not cause an afferent papillary defect. It may, however, blunt the red reflex and cause nystagmus or strabismus.

2. b. Diabetes causes refractive error shifts by changing the refractive index of the crystalline lens.

3. c. In general, the more anterior the opacity lies along the visual axis within the crystalline lens, the less effect will the opacity have on visual acuity.

4. c. The phenothiazines are antipsychotic medications (Haldol, Mellaril) that can cause corneal pigmentary deposits, macular pigment changes, and anterior subcapsular cataracts.

5. d. Angle recession represents widening of the anterior chamber angle due to trauma to the globe and may be seen by the clinician in association with lens subluxation in such cases; however, angle recession is not caused by lens subluxation.

6. d. Nuclear sclerotic lens changes are responsible for myopic shifts in refraction.

7. a. Steroid use can lead to posterior subcapsular cataract formation.

8. b. Specular reflection is typically used to evaluate the corneal endothelium. The other techniques are necessary for complete assessment of the crystalline lens when considering surgery.

9. c. Diabetic individuals have a significantly higher incidence of cortical cataract formation. Other cataract types can certainly be observed as well.

10. a. Hypermature cataract is the only type of cataract that typically causes zonular dehiscence; trauma and homocystinuria are causes as well, and it is this zonular breakdown that causes phacodonesis. High myopia alone is not a cause of phacodonesis because it does not cause a change in lens zonules.

11. a. Posterior subcapsular cataract development is a well-documented side effect of oral prednisone.

12. b. Leaking lens proteins from a hypermature cataract lead to phacolytic uveitis.

13. d. Stromal edema can signal the presence of herpes simplex keratitis or other corneal infection; active blepharitis is a risk factor for endophthalmitis following surgery; and a preexisting bleb could be compromised by the inflammatory response following surgery. Therefore, punctate epitheliopathy is the most benign finding listed.

14. d. Hyperopic individuals tend to have short eyes with lower axial lengths. The crystalline lens swelling that is often associated with cataract formation will crowd the angle the most in these patients, leading to an increase in intraocular pressure (IOP).

15. c. Keratometry is most needed before cataract surgery because this value is used in nomograms to calculate the correct IOL power. The other items listed have significantly less impact on the success of cataract surgery.

16. a. Subluxation of the lens can occur with Marfan's syndrome due to defective (stretched or broken) zonules. The subluxation is usually upward and temporal.

17. d. Posterior subcapsular cataracts have the greatest effect on vision when the pupil is small. Under those conditions, the cataracts are able to block most of the light entering the eye, whereas much more light gets around the central cataract when the pupil is larger.

18. b. It is believed that the greater capacity for lens epithelial cells to proliferate after surgery in younger patients results in less incidence of opacity in older patients. Iris pigment has nothing to do with formation of posterior capsular opacification. Polishing the capsule may help to prevent this complication but often is ineffective. YAG lasers are used in treatment to perform capsulotomy.

CHAPTER 23

Uveitis, Sclera/Episclera

Jennifer A. Palombi, Brad M. Sutton

1. All of the following are true of simple episcleritis EXCEPT:
   a. the patient will have marked injection
   b. pain may be absent
   c. there is often mucus discharge
   d. redness is often sectoral

2. All of the following are true of nodular episcleritis EXCEPT:
   a. nodules may be single or multiple
   b. nodules may undergo necrosis
   c. nodules can be moved over underlying sclera
   d. it tends to be localized to one part of the globe

3. Unilateral facial pigmentation accompanied by blue sclera on the same side is most common in which race?
   a. Caucasians
   b. Asians
   c. African-Americans
   d. Hispanics

4. A scleral condition requiring medical referral would be:
   a. episcleritis
   b. icteric sclera
   c. hyaline plaques
   d. nevus

5. Axenfeld's loops are:
   a. blue/black ciliary nerve loops on the scleral surface
   b. arteriovenous malformations
   c. more common in Caucasians
   d. most often found in the fornix

6.   A nevus of Ota is a(an) _____ condition.
     a.   malignant
     b.   autoimmune
     c.   unilateral
     d.   painful

7.   Blue sclera can be identified with all of the following conditions
     EXCEPT:
     a.   Marfan's syndrome
     b.   Paget's disease
     c.   Ehlers-Danlos syndrome
     d.   rheumatoid arthritis

8.   Hyaline plaques are:
     a.   common in children
     b.   a unilateral condition
     c.   sometimes associated with severe collagen vascular disease
     d.   the result of a toxicity reaction

9.   Icteric sclera is also known as:
     a.   pink eye
     b.   jaundice
     c.   blue sclera
     d.   melanosis

10. All of the following are true regarding scleromalacia perforans
     EXCEPT:
     a.   always occurs in the elderly
     b.   bulging occurs in the ectatic area
     c.   has no associated inflammation
     d.   develops slowly as a necrotic scleral thinning

11. Which of the following is an appropriate treatment for scleromalacia
     perforans?
     a.   subconjunctival steroids
     b.   topical steroids
     c.   high-dose systemic steroids
     d.   lubricants as needed

12. Staphyloma is defined as:
     a.   bulging of uveal tissue through thinning sclera
     b.   malignancy of the scleral tissue
     c.   benign tumor of the sclera
     d.   staphylococcal infection of the sclera

13. Which of the following is NOT a treatment for simple episcleritis?
   a. topical steroids
   b. topical vasoconstrictors
   c. systemic NSAIDs
   d. topical antibiotics

14. The nodule in nodular scleritis is a(an):
   a. fluid-filled cyst
   b. benign tumor
   c. area of cellular infiltrate
   d. trapped foreign body

15. Which of the following is NOT a clinical sign or symptom of scleritis?
   a. reduced vision
   b. photophobia
   c. severe pain
   d. minimal inflammation

16. Which of the following systemic conditions is commonly associated with scleritis?
   a. diabetes
   b. coronary artery disease
   c. systemic lupus erythematosus (SLE)
   d. acute anemia

17. A patient presenting with scleritis has a(an) _____ likelihood of having associated systemic disease.
   a. minimal (<2%)
   b. 10%
   c. 25%
   d. >50%
   e. absolute (100%)

18. Which of the following treatments is contraindicated in the treatment of scleritis?
   a. sub-Tenon's steroidal injection
   b. narcotic analgesia
   c. topical prednisone
   d. oral prednisone

19. Anterior uveitis may be subdivided into:
   a. iritis and iridocyclitis
   b. vitritis and pars planitis
   c. retinitis and choroiditis
   d. neither a, b, nor c

20. _____ involves inflammation of the choroid and retina posterior to the vitreous base.
   a. anterior uveitis
   b. posterior uveitis
   c. intermediate uveitis
   d. panuveitis

21. _____ affects the middle portion containing the ciliary body, vitreous, and retina.
   a. anterior uveitis
   b. posterior uveitis
   c. intermediate uveitis
   d. panuveitis

22. _____ is the classification given to inflammation affecting multiple parts of the same eye.
   a. anterior uveitis
   b. posterior uveitis
   c. intermediate uveitis
   d. panuveitis

23. Which of the following is most likely to present with bilateral uveitis?
   a. HLA-B27–associated uveitis
   b. toxocariasis
   c. Fuchs' iridocyclitis
   d. Vogt-Koyanagi-Harada syndrome

24. Uveitis can be classified as granulomatous if _____ is(are) present.
   a. mutton-fat KPs
   b. anterior chamber cells
   c. corneal infiltrates
   d. a confirmed diagnosis of underlying granulomatous systemic disease

25. The pain of iritis is generally attributable to:
   a. elevated IOP
   b. ciliary spasm
   c. retinal inflammation
   d. proptosis

26. Which of the following is useful in relieving the pain of iritis?
   a. topical steroids
   b. topical cycloplegics
   c. topical antibiotics
   d. topical NSAIDs

27. Which of the following is NOT a typical symptom of uveitis?
    a. pain
    b. photophobia
    c. mucus discharge
    d. blurred vision

28. Keratic precipitates are:
    a. clusters of inflammatory cells on the posterior corneal surface
    b. clusters of inflammatory cells floating in the anterior chamber
    c. exfoliative tissue floating in the posterior chamber
    d. exfoliative tissue on the posterior corneal surface

29. The cells of KPs arise from the:
    a. ciliary body
    b. aqueous humor
    c. vitreous
    d. pars plana

30. Generally, KPs from uveitis occur:
    a. on the inferior cornea
    b. on the superior cornea
    c. on the temporal cornea
    d. diffusely over the entire cornea

31. Anterior chamber flare is caused by:
    a. the formation of mutton fat KPs
    b. breakdown of the blood aqueous barrier
    c. corneal edema
    d. the presence of anterior chamber cells

32. A hypopyon is an accumulation of:
    a. protein
    b. leukocytes
    c. erythrocytes
    d. pigment

33. A hyphema is an accumulation of:
    a. protein
    b. leukocytes
    c. erythrocytes
    d. pigment

34. In assessing uveitis, masses on the iris at the pupillary border are called:
    a. Koeppe nodules
    b. Busacca nodules
    c. synechiae
    d. keratic precipitates

35. In assessing uveitis, masses on the anterior surface of the iris are called:
    a. Koeppe nodules
    b. Busacca nodules
    c. synechiae
    d. keratic precipitates

36. Busacca nodules are evidence of:
    a. retinitis
    b. panuveitis
    c. granulomatous uveitis
    d. nongranulomatous uveitis

37. Koeppe nodules are often located in areas that subsequently develop:
    a. iris atrophy
    b. anterior synechiae
    c. posterior synechiae
    d. persistent papillary membrane

38. If posterior synechiae formation proceeds unchecked during active uveitis, _____ may develop.
    a. pupillary block glaucoma
    b. cataract
    c. keratic precipitates
    d. acute angle closure glaucoma

39. If anterior synechiae formation proceeds unchecked during active uveitis, _____ may develop.
    a. pupillary block glaucoma
    b. cataract
    c. keratic precipitates
    d. acute angle closure glaucoma

40. Anterior stromal atrophy of the iris is characteristic of Fuchs' iridocyclitis and often results in _____.
    a. increased cells and flare
    b. transillumination defect
    c. heterochromia
    d. papillary block glaucoma

41. A frequent cause of decreased vision in anterior, intermediate, and posterior uveitis is:
    a. nuclear sclerotic lens changes
    b. cystoid macular edema
    c. vitreous haze
    d. optic neuropathy

42. In regard to retinal vasculitis, patients with sarcoid uveitis commonly have extensive _____, whereas patients with Behçet's disease tend to have more _____.
    a. phlebitis, arteritis
    b. arteritis, phlebitis
    c. phlebitis, crossing changes
    d. arteritis, crossing changes

43. Which of the following systemic conditions is most likely to cause a posterior uveitis (retinitis)?
    a. Still's disease
    b. ankylosing spondylitis
    c. toxoplasmosis
    d. Reiter's syndrome

44. Erythrocyte sedimentation rate (ESR) is an indicator of _____.
    a. systemic inflammatory activity
    b. rheumatoid factor
    c. systemic infection
    d. impaired coagulation

45. The serum ACE (angiotensin-converting enzyme) concentration is probably a reflection of the total amount of _____ in the body.
    a. white blood cells
    b. viral activity
    c. granulomatous tissue
    d. systemic inflammatory activity

46. Which of the following causes of uveitis is likely to cause an elevated ACE level?
    a. ankylosing spondylitis
    b. amyloidosis
    c. sarcoidosis
    d. rheumatoid arthritis

47. Which of the following causes of uveitis is NOT an HLA-associated disease?
    a. Behçet's disease
    b. ankylosing spondylitis
    c. Reiter's syndrome
    d. sarcoidosis

48. A 37-year-old man presents with active iridocyclitis accompanied by symptoms of pain and stiffness in the spine and limited chest expansion. A likely systemic etiology is:
    a. sarcoidosis
    b. ankylosing spondylitis
    c. rheumatoid arthritis
    d. Reiter's syndrome

49. In the treatment of anterior uveitis, topical steroids should be:
    a. tapered slowly to avoid rebound
    b. discontinued after the first week of treatment
    c. tapered as rapidly as possible to avoid side effects
    d. avoided—they are contraindicated

50. Which form of uveitis generally has little or no symptoms and must be diagnosed objectively?
    a. iritis
    b. iridocyclitis
    c. retinitis
    d. pars planitis

51. Which of the following is NOT significant in the diagnosis of chronic uveitis?
    a. vision
    b. bilaterality
    c. presence of KPs
    d. systemic disease

52. How is pain generally classified by a patient with acute anterior uveitis?
    a. foreign body sensation
    b. mild generalized headache
    c. deep, boring pain
    d. nonpainful

53. When should laboratory/medical testing be initiated for a patient presenting with uveitis?
    a. on the first occurrence
    b. on the second occurrence
    c. on the third occurrence
    d. after 1 year of recurrent episodes
    e. laboratory and medical testing is not indicated

54. Palliative care for a patient with acute anterior uveitis might include all of the following EXCEPT:
    a. dark glasses
    b. topical homatropine
    c. oral aspirin or ibuprofen
    d. antibiotics

55. A patient has presented with and begun initial therapy for acute anterior uveitis. This patient should be rechecked in:
    a. 24 to 48 hours
    b. 72 hours
    c. 1 week
    d. 2 weeks

56. Which of the following is an associated sign/symptom of Vogt-Koyanagi-Harada syndrome?
    a. positive chest x-ray
    b. vitiligo
    c. lymphadenopathy
    d. cramping and diarrhea

57. Which of the following is an associated sign/symptom of Crohn's disease?
    a. positive chest x-ray
    b. vitiligo
    c. lymphadenopathy
    d. cramping and diarrhea

58. Which of the following is an associated sign/symptom of sarcoidosis?
    a. positive chest x-ray
    b. vitiligo
    c. lymphadenopathy
    d. cramping and diarrhea

59. Which of the following is an associated sign/symptom of mononucleosis?
    a. positive chest x-ray
    b. vitiligo
    c. lymphadenopathy
    d. cramping and diarrhea

60. All of the following are blood tests to be ordered in the diagnosis of chronic uveitis EXCEPT:
    a. VDRL (venereal disease research lab)
    b. FTA-ABS (fluorescein treponema antibody-absorption)
    c. WBC (white blood cell count)
    d. HbA_{1C} (hemoglobin A_{1C})

Answers

1. c. There is no mucus discharge with episcleritis. There may be slight watering.

2. b. No necrosis occurs in episcleritis.

3. b. The condition, nevus of Ota, is most common in Asians.

4. b. Icteric sclera. A person with jaundice should be referred for further medical evaluation.

5. a. Axenfeld's loops are blue/black nerve loops on the scleral surface. They are most common in African-Americans and usually found within a few millimeters of the limbus.

6. c. A nevus of Ota has a unilateral presentation. It is a macular lesion on the side of the face involving the conjunctiva and lids, as well as the adjacent facial skin, sclera, ocular muscles, and periosteum.

7. d. Blue sclera is not typically associated with rheumatoid arthritis.

8. c. Hyaline plaques are sometimes associated with collagen vascular disease.

9. b. Icteric sclera is the clinical term for jaundice manifested as a yellowing of the sclera.

10. c. There is no associated bulge with scleral thinning from scleromalacia perforans.

11. c. High-dose systemic steroids are indicated for the treatment of scleromalacia perforans. Subconjunctival steroids are highly contraindicated, and topical agents are not beneficial.

12. a. Staphyloma is defined as a bulging of uveal tissue through thinning sclera.

13. d. Simple episcleritis is not infectious and does not require topical antibiotic therapy.

14. c. The nodule in nodular scleritis is an organized area of cellular infiltrate.

15. d. Inflammation with scleritis is often pronounced.

16. c. Scleritis is often associated with rheumatoid disease, including SLE.

17. d. A patient presenting with scleritis has a >50% likelihood of having associated systemic disease.

18. a. Sub-Tenon's or subconjunctival steroidal injections are contraindicated for scleritis.

19. a. Anterior uveitis refers to inflammation of the iris alone or the iris and ciliary body; anterior uveitis is the most common form. Inflammation of the iris may appropriately be termed iritis, whereas inflammation of the iris and the ciliary body is called iridocyclitis.

20. b. Posterior uveitis is inflammation of the choroids. Posterior uveitis is a vision disorder characterized by inflammation of the layer of blood vessels underlying the retina, and usually of the retina as well.

21. c. Intermediate uveitis is characterized by involvement of the ciliary body (pars plana), the extreme periphery of the retina, and the underlying choroid.

22. d. Panuveitis includes all parts of the uvea. When *inflammation* is located in multiple parts of the same eye (anterior, intermediate, and posterior sections), it is classified as panuveitis.

23. d. Vogt-Koyanagi-Harada syndrome often presents with bilateral uveitis.

24. a. Mutton-fat KPs, vitreous snowballs, and choroidal granulomas are all signs of granulomatous uveitis.

25. b. Ciliary spasm is the primary source of pain in iritis.

26. b. Topical cycloplegics are useful for relieving iritis pain because they quiet ciliary spasm.

27. c. Mucus discharge is not associated with uveitis. The patient may complain of watery discharge due to excess tearing from photophobia.

28. a. Keratic precipitates are clusters of inflammatory cells on the endothelial surface of the cornea.

29. b. Cells from KPs arise from the aqueous humor.

30. a. The most common distribution of KPs is on the inferior cornea.

31. b. Flare is caused by the breakdown of the blood-aqueous barrier and subsequent release of protein.

32. b. A hypopyon is an accumulation of leukocytes.

33. c. A hyphema is an accumulation of erythrocytes.

34. a. Masses on the iris at the pupillary border are called Koeppe nodules.

35. b. In assessing uveitis, masses on the anterior surface of the iris are called Busacca nodules.

36. c. Busacca nodules are evidence of granulomatous inflammation.

37. c. Koeppe nodules are often located at sites that subsequently develop posterior synechiae.

38. a. If posterior synechiae formation proceeds unchecked, pupillary block glaucoma may develop.

39. d. If anterior synechiae formation proceeds unchecked during active uveitis, acute angle closure glaucoma may develop.

40. c. Anterior stromal atrophy of the iris is characteristic of Fuchs' iridocyclitis and often results in heterochromia.

41. b. CME may contribute to decreased vision in all forms of uveitis and should be ruled out by dilated fundus examination.

42. a. In regard to retinal vasculitis, patients with sarcoid uveitis commonly have extensive phlebitis (vasculitis of the veins), whereas patients with Behçet's disease tend to have more arteritis (vasculitis of the arteries).

43. c. Toxoplasmosis often causes retinitis, whereas the other choices tend to cause iritis (anterior uveitis).

44. a. ESR measures systemic inflammatory activity.

45. c. The serum ACE concentration is probably a reflection of the total amount of granulomatous tissue in the body.

46. b. Amyloidosis causes an elevated ACE level on laboratory testing.

47. d. Sarcoidosis is a rheumatoid disease.

48. b. Ankylosing spondylitis is characterized by inflammatory stiffening of the spine and rib cage through calcification of the nonsynovial (cartilaginous) synchondrosis of the intervertebral spaces.

49. a. Topical steroids should be very slowly tapered to avoid rebound of the inflammation.

50. d. Pars planitis generally has little subjective symptomatology.

51. a. Vision may be normal in uveitis and therefore is not an indicator of chronic disease.

52. c. Anterior uveitis is generally associated with deep, boring pain.

53. b. Laboratory and medical testing is indicated to rule out an underlying systemic medial condition after the second occurrence of uveitis.

54. d. Antibiotics will have no effect on the pain of uveitis.

55. a. A patient begun on therapy for acute uveitis should be rechecked in 24 to 48 hours to check for efficacy and side effects of the treatment.

56. b. An associated symptom of VKH is vitiligo. Vitiligo manifests in over 50% of patients and is often symmetric. Most patients have perilimbal vitiligo (Sugiura sign). VKH syndrome is a systemic risk factor for uveitis.

57. d. An associated symptom of Crohn's disease is cramping and diarrhea. Some people with Crohn's disease have minor symptoms and little discomfort or pain. Their symptoms may only occur a few times. But others may experience frequent diarrhea, intestinal ulcers, and problems in other parts of their bodies, such as inflammation of the joints, skin rashes, and eye problems. Crohn's is a systemic risk factor for uveitis.

58. a. Positive chest x-ray. Sarcoidosis is an inflammatory condition of unknown etiology that can affect any part of the body, particularly the lungs, lymph nodes in the chest, skin, and eyes. About 25% to 50% of patients with sarcoidosis will be found to have ocular disease. Sarcoidosis is a systemic risk factor for uveitis.

59. c. Lymphadenopathy is an associated sign for mononucleosis.
Mononucleosis is a systemic risk factor for uveitis.

60. d. HbA_{1C} is a laboratory test for diabetes.

Retina/Vitreous

Leo P. Semes

1. Which of the following is/are NOT true of the foveal avascular zone?
   a. entirely supplied by the choriocapillaris
   b. approximately 1 DD (disk diameter) in normals
   c. shows up as a dark area on fluorescein angiography because the RPE cells are more columnar in shape and contain more pigment granules to block the choroidal fluorescence
   d. contains no retinal blood vessels

2. Which of the following circulatory systems supplies the nerve fiber layer?
   a. choroidal
   b. retinal
   c. neither
   d. both

3. Which of the following is NOT true of sodium fluorescein?
   a. stains skin and mucous membranes yellowish for up to a day and a half
   b. is eliminated through liver and kidneys
   c. may contaminate laboratory tests for up to 5 days
   d. contained in red blood cells rather than in serum

4. B-scan ultrasonography is most valuable in cases of unilateral reduced vision and:
   a. opaque media
   b. clear media
   c. either opaque or clear media
   d. a need for cataract surgery

5. The best description of the clinical information gained from OCT (optical coherence tomography) would be:
   a. elucidation of tissue depth for localization
   b. cross-sectional tissue imaging (in vivo histology)
   c. localization by three-dimensional imaging from A-scan reconstruction
   d. topographic representation of the macula

6. In which of the following would you perform or order B-scan ultrasound?
   a. unilateral traumatic cataract preventing visualization of the posterior pole
   b. nerve head drusen that you identify at slit-lamp biomicroscopy
   c. suspected macular hole with positive Watzke-Allen sign
   d. all of the above

7. CSME occurs in which of the following clinical presentations?
   a. mild NPDR (nonproliferative diabetic retinopathy)
   b. moderate NPDR
   c. mild PDR (proliferative diabetic retinopathy)
   d. high-risk PDR
   e. CSME can occur in any of the above

8. Which of the following treatments would be applied in diabetic NVD?
   a. vitrectomy
   b. intravitreal triamcinolone acetonide injection
   c. membrane peel
   d. panretinal photocoagulation

9. Venous beading is NOT characteristic of which of the following stages of NPDR?
   a. mild
   b. moderate
   c. severe
   d. very severe

10. Which of the following is NOT true of IRMA?
    a. develops near zones of capillary nonperfusion
    b. develops within the framework of existing vessel network
    c. acts to shunt blood around a closed area in vaso-occlusive disorders
    d. occurs only at the disc

11. IRMA is the acronym for:
    a. intraretinal microvascular abnormalities
    b. international retinal micron aberrations
    c. intracapillary microaneurysms
    d. intravitreal retinal microaneurysms

12. The color of the sensory retina is:
    a. red-orange
    b. black
    c. transparent
    d. yellow-orange
    e. varies depending on RPE density and choroidal pigmentation

13. PDT (photodynamic therapy) can be applied to other subfoveal disorders. Which of the following would not be amenable to PDT treatment?
    a. ocular histoplasmosis with macular involvement
    b. CSME (central serous macular edema) in diabetic retinopathy
    c. pathologic myopia with subfoveal lesion
    d. angioid streaks with choroidal neovascularization

14. Laser photocoagulation has application to all of the following EXCEPT:
    a. diabetic CSME (central serous macular edema)
    b. diabetic NVE (neovascularization elsewhere)
    c. retinal tears prior to scleral buckling
    d. macular hole repair
    e. juxtafoveal and extrafoveal CNVM (choroidal neovascular membrane)

15. PDT (photodynamic therapy) has been shown to have application in which of the following?
    a. subfoveal CNVM (choroidal neovascular membrane)
    b. pathologic myopia
    c. ocular histoplasmosis syndrome
    d. angioid streaks
    e. all of the above may be amenable to PDT

16. Which of the following pigmented fundus lesions is most likely to have a systemic connection?
    a. malignant melanoma
    b. melanocytoma
    c. CHRPE (congenital hypertrophy of the retinal pigment epithelium)
    d. choroidal nevus
    e. all of the above

17. Clinical evaluation (standard of care) for patients taking chloroquine (or hydroxychloroquine) includes all of the following EXCEPT:
    a. ultrasonography or OCT imaging
    b. dark adaptation
    c. VF (visual field; central 10°)
    d. color vision evaluation
    e. photographic documentation

18. Which of the following is a primary retinitis (as opposed to a primary choroiditis)?
    a. histoplasmosis
    b. toxoplasmosis
    c. toxocariasis
    d. malignant choroidal melanoma
    e. they are all interchangeable

19. The only pigmented tumor of the optic nerve head is:
    a. melanocytoma
    b. astrocytoma
    c. retinoblastoma
    d. glioma
    e. glaucoma

20. Which of the following would NOT be associated with AION (anterior ischemic optic neuropathy)?
    a. potentially caused by optic nerve drusen
    b. usually has ischemic etiology and consequences
    c. shows altitudinal visual field defect
    d. managed with oral steroids
    e. diabetes is a major systemic risk factor

21. Which of the following observations is consistent with acute papilledema?
    a. hemorrhages
    b. exudates
    c. dilated blood vessels
    d. only a and c
    e. all of the above

22. Which is NOT characterized by a swollen or elevated optic nerve?
    a. papilledema
    b. optic disc drusen
    c. RBON (retrobulbar optic neuritis)
    d. papillitis
    e. metastasis to the optic nerve

23. Which of the following is/are a component(s) of Bactrim?
    a. sulfamethoxazole
    b. trimethoprim
    c. bacitracin
    d. both a and b
    e. both b and c

24. The signature clinical evidence of PVD is:
    a. positive Watzke-Allen sign (test)
    b. negative Watzke-Allen sign
    c. Weiss ring observation
    d. presence of lacunae
    e. absence of Weiss ring

25. The weakest attachment between the vitreous and retina is:
    a. at the vitreous base
    b. at the vitreous apex
    c. at the posterior pole
    d. around the macula
    e. fine fibrils throughout the vitreoretinal interface

26. Which of the following is/are NOT predisposing to retinal detachment?
    a. lattice retinal degeneration
    b. retinoschisis
    c. pavingstone degeneration
    d. asymptomatic retinal break
    e. symptomatic retinal break

27. Histopathologically, the SRF surround of a retinal break is located between:
    a. NFL and GCL
    b. PRL and RPE
    c. RPE and Bruch membrane
    d. Bruch membrane and choroid

28. Which of the following is NOT consistent with all lattice lesions?
    a. branching white lines
    b. adherent vitreous surrounding the lesion
    c. liquefied vitreous within the lesion
    d. loss of inner retinal layers

29. Your patient is 14 years old. Which of the following conditions would you be most likely to observe when performing fundus evaluation?
    a. reticular midperipheral pigment degeneration (tapetochoroidal degeneration)
    b. lattice
    c. pavingstone degeneration
    d. cystoid degeneration
    e. cystic retinal tuft

30. In which of the following cases would you expect stability after the age of 20?
    a. reticular midperipheral pigment degeneration (tapetochoroidal degeneration)
    b. lattice degeneration
    c. pavingstone degeneration
    d. cystic retinal tuft

31. Contemporary management of lattice consists of:
    a. uniform prophylaxis
    b. prophylaxis based on refractive correction and age
    c. observation with prophylaxis recommendation based on specific risk factors
    d. scleral buckle

32. The major distinction for recommending prophylaxis in predisposing conditions to RD (retinal detachment) is:
    a. symptoms
    b. lattice
    c. PVD (posterior vitreal detachment)
    d. impending intraocular surgery
    e. diabetes

33. Regarding the signs and symptoms of rhegmatogenous retinal detachment secondary to PVD (posterior vitreal detachment), which of the following is/are most predictive?
    a. breaks generally develop within 6 weeks when symptomatic
    b. presence of both flashes and floaters is stronger than either alone
    c. both a and b are true
    d. breaks are present in only 50% of PVDs

34. Which of the following would most likely appear in the vertical meridians?
    a. lattice/short posterior ciliary nerves
    b. lattice/long posterior ciliary nerves
    c. cystoid degeneration/pavingstone degeneration
    d. tapetochoroidal degeneration/lattice

35. In which of the following conditions would the histopathologic change involve the choriocapillaris?
    a. lattice degeneration
    b. pavingstone degeneration
    c. tapetochoroidal degeneration
    d. retinoschisis
    e. retinal detachment

36. Clinically, which of the following would most resemble RP?
    a. peripheral tapetochoroidal degeneration
    b. lattice degeneration
    c. pavingstone degeneration
    d. cystoid degeneration
    e. retinoschisis

37. Which of the following does NOT involve inner retinal layers?
    a. cystic retinal tuft
    b. lattice degeneration
    c. symptomatic linear retinal break (tear)
    d. tapetochoroidal degeneration

38. Remodeled pigment in the retina could be a sign of which of the following?
    a. inflammation
    b. infection
    c. vitreoretinal traction
    d. only a and b
    e. a, b, and c

39. Your patient is a 62-year-old black woman with congenital "toxo" scars in the macula (VA = 20/400). You observe reactivation equatorially in the right fundus. Proper management is:
    a. fight to preserve vision with aggressive antibiotic therapy (e.g., Bactrim)
    b. refer for fluorescein angiography and prophylactic treatment
    c. monitor in 2 to 4 weeks
    d. warn the patient of signs and symptoms of RD and recheck in 3 months

40. The proximate cause of most (95%) retinal detachments (rhegmatogenous) is:
    a. lattice retinal degeneration
    b. posterior vitreous detachment
    c. linear retinal breaks
    d. choroidal malignant melanoma
    e. trauma

41. Asteroid bodies are present in patients without symptoms and (generally) without systemic conditions. Which of the following pairs of statements is true?
    a. unilateral in about three fourths of cases and move with eye movements
    b. usually bilateral and interfere with fundus evaluation
    c. usually unilateral and associated with diabetes in >50% of cases
    d. age related and represent a precursor to AMD

42. The contemporary view of MH (macular hole) evolution includes all of the following EXCEPT:
    a. anterior-posterior vitreous traction
    b. perimacular PVD (posterior vitreal detachment)
    c. foveal cyst formation
    d. radial forces that enlarge an incipient hole
    e. operculum formation at stage 2 or 3

43. Which of the following is a symptom of macular hole?
    a. positive W-A finding
    b. distinctive image on OCT
    c. both a and b
    d. reduced VA
    e. any of the above

44. The course (prognosis/outcome) for macular holes is dependent on which of the following?
    a. later stage (poorer prognosis)
    b. initial VA (better VA is better prognosis)
    c. fresher is better
    d. all of the above are dependent factors for MH outcome

45. Which of the following is a protozoan (obligate intracellular parasite)?
    a. *Treponema pallidium*
    b. *Bartonella henselae*
    c. *Toxoplasmosis gondii*
    d. *Histoplasma capsulatum*
    e. *Staphylococcus aureus*

46. Contemporary treatment of "ocular toxo" may include all of the following EXCEPT:
    a. clindamycin
    b. Bactrim
    c. azithromycin
    d. atovaquone
    e. pyrimethamine + triple sulf

47. Lesions large enough to fill a condensing lens may be suspicious for malignancy. What other characteristic would be attributable to malignant or suspicious fundus lesion?
    a. elevation
    b. drusen on the surface
    c. subclinical retinal detachment
    d. either a or c

Answers

1. b. The FAZ (foveal avascular zone) is only about 1/3 DD but is supplied by the choroidal circulation and is free of retinal capillaries.

2. d. The inner retinal is supplied by branches of the central retinal artery.

3. d. Fluorescein is water soluble and is mixed in the serum but does not combine with red blood cells.

4. a. Observation in full color and three dimensions is preferable to one dimension in black and white. B-scan is the later presentation and is most useful when the fundus cannot be directly visualized.

5. b. This relatively new technology utilizes A-scan to represent retinal layers in a cross-sectional presentation that shows a false-color "histological" picture of retinal layers and vitreoretinal interface.

6. a. OCT (optical coherence tomography) would be valuable for macular hole, and direct visualization of ONH (optic nerve head) drusen would be sufficient for diagnosis, but opaque media would be the greatest call for using B-scan imaging.

7. e. CSME is independent of the stage of diabetic retinopathy and whether it is proliferative or nonproliferative.

8. d. Neovascularization (NV) is a response to hypoxia, and when portions of the retina are destroyed, this demand is reduced, thus reducing the stimulus to NV.

9. a. The distinguishing characteristics of progression of nonproliferative DR are venous beading and IRMA. These are not present in the early (mild) stage.

10. d. IRMA represents retinal capillary dropout and as such will not occur at the optic disc. The channels of enlarged blood vessels of IRMA become evident clinically and shunt blood around the deficient capillary beds.

11. a. Self-explanatory.

12. c. The sensory retina would be nonfunctional if it were any color. The clinician should keep in mind that the photoreceptors are part of the outer retina and lie beneath the NFL and other components of the inner retina. The characteristic fundus appearance is due to the underlying RPE, choroidal vasculature, and pigmentation.

13. b. Diabetic CSME does not involve new vessel formation and therefore would not be a consideration for PDT treatment.

14. d. Macular hole repair is effected via vitrectomy and membrane peel while the others may be treated (a) focally, (b) with panretinal, or (c) as a posterior barrier to progression.

15. e. Neovascular processes, even those involving the center of the macula, are being shown to have application and efficacy from PDT.

16. c. Among these, melanocytoma and CHRPE are congenital. Malignant melanoma (MM) and choroidal nevus are probably acquired, and rarely is MM from metastasis. CHRPE has been reported to have various prevalences among patients with Gardner's syndrome and familiar polyposis.

17. a. Recent guidelines for chloroquine retinopathy evaluation include structural evaluation and functional testing but not objective imaging with OCT.

18. a. *Histoplasma capsulatum* primarily attacks the choroidal vasculature. Secondarily there is retinal involvement. The toxos are primarily retinal in involvement, whereas malignant melanoma is not inflammatory (i.e., not an "-itis.")

19. a. Astrocytoma is tapioca colored and associated with neurofibromatosis; retinoblastoma is one of the etiologies in leukocoria; glioma involves neural tissue and is lightly if at all colored; and glaucoma is not a tumor.

20. d. Oral steroids would be indicated in giant cell arteritis.

21. e. The typical picture of acute papilledema is one of hemorrhage, exudate, and dilated blood vessels.

22. c. In retrobulbar optic neuritis, the characteristic clinical findings are that the doctor sees nothing and the patient sees nothing. The optic disc looks normal but the patient has reduced vision.

23. d. Bactrim is sulfamethoxazole and trimethoprim.

24. c. Weiss ring is the putative sign of PVD. This represents the
         clinical evidence of release of attachment of the vitreous from
         the optic disc.

25. e. The strongest attachments are at the base and posterior pole. The
         vitreous is weakly attached at the macula (normally) but only very
         weakly attached throughout the vitreous-retina interface.

26. c. Retinal breaks and lattice are well-known predisposing conditions
         to RD. Retinoschisis is rarely associated with RD, but pavingstone
         represents loss of outer retinal layers with consequent sealing of
         the remaining inner retina to the underlying Bruch membrane.

27. b. RD occurs between the RPE and the sensory retina, specifically the
         PRL.

28. a. Lattice is an inner retinal disorder that includes developmental
         changes of the vitreous and inner retina. Later, vitreous changes
         involving vitreovascular interaction develop, resulting in white
         lines.

29. d. Cystoid is present in all over the age of 8 years and has been reported
         in premature infants. Reticular degeneration and pavingstone are
         age-related findings. Lattice is discovered in patients most
         frequently between 10 and 20 years of age. Cystic tuft, although
         congenital, is present in only 8% of the population.

30. b. Reticular and pavingstone are age related and rarely occur before
         age 40 years. Cystic tuft may evolve into opercular hole with PVD,
         usually after the age of 40 years.

31. c. Only one lattice lesion in 100 will result in RD.

32. a. It has been well documented that symptomatic patients (flashes/
         floaters) are the best candidates (at greatest risk of RD).

33. c. This has been well documented in two studies from the
         Netherlands and Great Britain.

34. a. Anatomically, the SPC nerves are located on either side of the
         vertical meridians, and lattice has been documented to occur most
         frequently (by far) vertically.

35. b. Histopathological studies of pavingstone show that the underlying
         choriocapillaris is regionally impacted, leaving the overlying RPE
         without a nutritional source. The RPE migrates to the edges, where
         anastomoses offer available nutrition.

36.   a.   The only generalized pigmented change among those listed is in tapetochoroidal degeneration.

37.   d.   As the name suggests, tapetochoroidal degeneration involves the outer retina and RPE.

38.   a.   Insults to the retina and underlying RPE result in remodeling of the RPE with resultant clinical manifestations. Etiologies include all of the three.

39.   c.   Because this patient has a macular lesion that has claimed the vision, even though the location per se would suggest treatment option, observation is the option most useful for this situation.

40.   b.   The proximity and adherence of the vitreous and retina throughout their mutual extent make PVD the obvious choice.

41.   a.   No systemic relationships have been established with asteroids. They are typically unilateral and attached to the framework of the vitreous, making them mobile with eye movements.

42.   d.   Previous theories of MH suggested enlargement in a radial pattern. Evidence from OCT has suggested that residual attachment at the macula following PVD and the anterior-posterior forces that act with eye movement are responsible for MH formation.

43.   d.   The first two are clinical findings; only reduced VA is a symptom.

44.   d.   These facts have been reported from imaging studies.

45.   c.   *Treponema pallidium, Staphylococcus aureus,* and *Bartonella henselae* are bacterial; *Histoplasma capsulatum* is fungal.

46.   e.   The classic (historical) treatment is triple sulfa; contemporary alternatives are clindamycin and azithromycin, with Bactrin as the treatment of choice.

47.   d.   Drusen are consistent with long-standing lesions, but elevation and SRF would signal growth, a key feature of malignant transformation.

Neuro-Ophthalmic Disease

Kelly A. Malloy

1. All of the following tests assess the afferent visual system function EXCEPT:
    a. color vision
    b. cover test
    c. swinging flashlight test
    d. visual field test

2. If the patient has an evident unilateral visual field defect, with no evidence of relative afferent pupillary defect or dyschromatopsia, the LEAST LIKELY etiology is:
    a. glaucoma
    b. macular degeneration
    c. nonglaucomatous optic neuropathy
    d. focal retinal detachment

3. A CT scan is superior to an MRI for which of the following?
    a. suspected bleeding
    b. suspected bone fracture
    c. both a and b
    d. a CT scan is never superior to an MRI

4. All of the following would be contraindications to having an MRI EXCEPT:
    a. pacemaker
    b. metallic foreign body in orbit
    c. weight above 400 pounds
    d. pregnancy because of radiation exposure

5. MRA would be used to look for all of the following EXCEPT:
    a. venous sinus thrombosis
    b. arteriovenous malformation
    c. aneurysm
    d. carotid artery dissection

6. A right abduction deficit with decreased sensation in the distribution of V1 and V2 on the right side localizes to the:
   a. abducens nucleus
   b. pons
   c. subarachnoid space
   d. right cavernous sinus

7. A cecocentral scotoma indicates damage to which of the following?
   a. papillomacular nerve fiber bundle
   b. arcuate nerve fiber bundle
   c. nasal nerve fiber bundle
   d. none of the above

8. All of the following are considered emergent clinical presentations, requiring immediate work-up/hospitalization/treatment EXCEPT:
   a. right-sided ptosis, miosis, and neck pain
   b. bilateral optic swelling, headache, pulsatile tinnitus, and lack of spontaneous venous pulse
   c. reversing hyperdeviation with fixed, dilated pupil in eye that is higher in downgaze
   d. bilateral proptosis, eyelid retraction, and lid lag

9. All of the following visual field defects could occur with a lesion of the posterior aspect of the optic chiasm EXCEPT:
   a. central bitemporal visual field defect
   b. central scotoma with superior temporal defect in contralateral eye
   c. bitemporal hemianopia denser inferiorly
   d. incongruous homonymous hemianopia

10. All of the following visual field defects localize to the visual cortex (occipital lobe) EXCEPT:
    a. temporal crescent sparing
    b. temporal crescent involvement
    c. foveal/macular sparing
    d. central homonymous hemianopia

11. Optic disc pallor can occur from lesions of all of the following EXCEPT:
    a. optic nerve
    b. optic chiasm
    c. lateral geniculate
    d. optic radiations

12. Optochoroidal shunt vessels can occur with all of the following EXCEPT:
    a. sphenoid wing meningioma
    b. glaucoma
    c. chronic papilledema
    d. traumatic optic neuropathy

13. Optic disc hemorrhages are LEAST LIKELY with which of the following?
    a. nonarteritic anterior ischemic optic neuropathy
    b. arteritic anterior ischemic optic neuropathy
    c. optic neuritis
    d. acute papilledema

14. Which region of the optic disc would be the LAST to swell in papilledema?
    a. nasal
    b. temporal
    c. superior
    d. inferior

15. All of the following could be associated with a hypoplastic optic disc EXCEPT:
    a. scleral ring around disc
    b. possible visual field defects
    c. possible association with central nervous system and endocrine abnormalities
    d. always bilateral

16. Which is the LEAST LIKELY to be associated with pain?
    a. giant cell arteritis
    b. optic neuritis
    c. nonarteritic anterior ischemic optic neuropathy
    d. aneurysmal cranial nerve III palsy

17. All of the following are potential features of optic neuropathy EXCEPT:
    a. anisocoria
    b. reduced visual acuity
    c. red desaturation
    d. visual field loss

18. Which of the following does not cause a relative afferent pupillary defect in the involved eye?
    a. cataract
    b. ischemic optic neuropathy
    c. large retinal detachment
    d. optic neuritis

19. All of the following can have the feature of better pupillary reaction to accommodation than to light stimulus EXCEPT:
    a. a vasculopathic (diabetic) cranial nerve III palsy
    b. a compressive cranial nerve III palsy
    c. tonic pupil
    d. tectal pupil (dorsal midbrain syndrome)

20. All of the following could present as anisocoria, with the greater difference in pupil size in bright illumination, EXCEPT:
    a. an aneurysmal CN III palsy
    b. Adie's tonic pupil
    c. iris sphincter tears
    d. an oculosympathetic paresis
    e. ocular contamination from a scopolamine patch used for motion sickness

21. All of the following are consistent with oculosympathetic paresis (Horner syndrome) EXCEPT:
    a. ptosis
    b. inverse (upside-down) ptosis
    c. miosis
    d. aniscocoria greatest in dim illumination
    e. anisocoria greater at 12 seconds into darkness than 5 seconds into darkness

22. All of the following may potentially be needed to diagnose the cause of a Horner syndrome EXCEPT:
    a. MRI of brain
    b. MRA/angiogram of neck
    c. MRI of lumbar spine
    d. chest CT scan
    e. urine tests specific for neuroblastoma

23. You see a 2-year-old child with ptosis and miosis OD and heterochromia iridis with the right iris being lighter. The parents note that they first noticed the eyelid droop about 2 months ago. Which of the following is the MOST APPROPRIATE?
    a. it is congenital Horner's since heterochromia is present
    b. no work-up is needed
    c. only an MRI of the brain is needed
    d. the work-up may include imaging of the brain, abdomen, and chest, as well as urine tests

24. The following are true regarding the work-up/treatment of a suspected aneurysmal CN III palsy EXCEPT:
    a. patient needs an MRI and MRA
    b. patient may need an arteriogram
    c. this is an emergent situation
    d. you would expect spontaneous resolution within 3 months without treatment
    e. the concern is rupture of the aneurysm, leading to a subarachnoid hemorrhage

25. Vertical diplopia can be caused by all of the following EXCEPT:
    a. myasthenia gravis
    b. thyroid orbitopathy
    c. aneurysmal CN III palsy
    d. pseudotumor cerebri
    e. traumatic cranial nerve IV palsy

26. All of the following are true regarding cyclotorsion in a CN IV palsy EXCEPT:
    a. if objective excyclotorsion is present, the macula will appear to be rotated downward
    b. the diplopic patient will report the higher image to be tilted
    c. subjective excyclotorsion can be tested with double Maddox rod testing
    d. the superior oblique muscle, when fully functional, acts to intort the eye

27. Your patient sustained recent trauma and complains of vertical diplopia and tilted objects. You perform a double Maddox rod test and obtain 12 degrees of excyclotorsion. Which would be the LEAST LIKELY association?
    a. downward displacement of the macula
    b. esodeviation
    c. dorsal midbrain syndrome will be in the differential diagnosis
    d. a right hyper on right head tilt and a left hyper on left head tilt
    e. the symptoms will fully resolve in 3 months without the need for surgical correction

28. You are told that the patient in the figure below (in primary gaze) has a recent-onset cranial nerve IV palsy. You would expect to see all of the following EXCEPT:

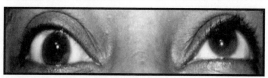

   a. Hyper worse in right gaze
   b. Hyper worse on right head tilt
   c. Subjective excyclotorsion
   d. Objective excyclotorsion

29. If an abduction deficit was caused by thyroid orbitopathy (restrictive), which would be LEAST LIKELY?
   a. slowed saccades (glissades)
   b. positive forced duction test
   c. infiltrated rectus muscle
   d. ductions are equal to versions

30. All of the following are consistent with myasthenia gravis EXCEPT:
   a. variable ptosis
   b. fatigable ptosis
   c. positive ice pack test
   d. anisocoria
   e. potential association of a thymoma

31. A bilateral inferior altitudinal visual field defect, in the setting of a normal appearing optic disc and retinal evaluation in each eye, is most likely associated with which of the following?
   a. bilateral NA-AION
   b. bilateral retinal abnormalities
   c. bilateral occipital lobe infarcts above the calcarine fissure
   d. bilateral parietal lobe infarcts

32. Your 32-year-old female patient reports a 3-day sudden vision loss and dyschromatopsia OD, along with pain on eye movements. You find 20/80 VA OD and a cecocentral scotoma OD. You would do all of the following EXCEPT:
   a. obtain an MRI
   b. start the patient on IV methylprednisolone
   c. start the patient on oral prednisone
   d. rule out Lyme disease
   e. consider immunomodulation treatment if there are multiple periventricular white matter changes on MRI

33. Which of the following is the single BEST factor in predicting which optic neuritis patient will go on to develop multiple sclerosis?
    a. MRI white matter lesions
    b. CSF-oligoclonal banding pattern
    c. severity of VA loss from optic neuritis
    d. birthplace (distance from equator)

34. All of the following could be features of congenital nystagmus EXCEPT:
    a. combination of pendular and jerk components to the nystagmus
    b. vertical nystagmus
    c. latent nystagmus
    d. presence of a null zone

35. Blood thinners can be an appropriate treatment for all of the following EXCEPT:
    a. carotid artery dissection
    b. stroke
    c. hemorrhagic stroke
    d. carotid artery stenosis

36. All of the following are potential aspects of the work-up for myasthenia gravis EXCEPT:
    a. chest CT scan
    b. acetylcholine receptor antibodies
    c. serum protein electrophoresis
    d. single-fiber electromyography (EMG)

37. Mestinon (pyridostigmine), an acetylcholine esterase inhibitor, is used as a treatment for which condition?
    a. Graves' disease
    b. myasthenia gravis
    c. multiple sclerosis
    d. Hashimoto's thyroiditis

38. The most common muscle to be involved in thyroid orbitopathy is:
    a. inferior rectus
    b. superior rectus
    c. medial rectus
    d. lateral rectus

39. If a right abduction deficit is present as a feature of thyroid orbitopathy, it is due to:
    a. infiltration of the belly of the right lateral rectus muscle
    b. infiltration of the belly of the right medial rectus muscle
    c. infiltration of the belly and tendons of the right lateral rectus muscle
    d. infiltration of the belly and tendons of the right medial rectus muscle

40. A gaze palsy on right gaze and an internuclear ophthalmoplegia on left gaze together would make up which of the following?
   a. skew deviation
   b. binocular internuclear ophthalmoplegia
   c. one-and-a-half syndrome
   d. Foville's syndrome

Answers

1. b. The cover test assesses the efferent visual system/ocular motility. The others are tests of optic nerve or afferent function.

2. c. A unilateral nonglaucomatous optic neuropathy will present with features of an RAPD and relative decrease in color saturation. Although minimal damage to the optic nerve will cause an RAPD and dyschromatopsia, it takes a significant amount of retinal damage to cause the same clinical findings.

3. c. Although MRI is preferred over CT for imaging of soft tissue structures, a CT scan is the test of choice for trauma. This is because CT is better at imaging both blood and bone and therefore would be better able to detect subtle bleeding and bone fractures.

4. d. MRI uses a magnetic field and therefore has no radiation exposure, as does a CT scan. However, the magnetic field is responsible for the MRI contraindications of pacemakers and metallic foreign bodies.

5. a. An MRA (magnetic resonance angiogram) is used to visualize the arterial circulation. Although the other three choices affect the arterial system, a venous sinus thrombosis occurs in the venous drainage system of the brain. Therefore, an MRV (magnetic resonance venogram) would be needed to image a venous sinus thrombosis.

6. d. The right CN VI, as well as the right V1 and V2 (along with the right CN III, IV, and sympathetics), travels in the right cavernous sinus. A lesion of the abducens nucleus would produce a gaze palsy, not an abduction deficit. A lesion of CN VI in the pons or subarachnoid space would not selectively affect CN V1 and V2.

7. a. A cecocentral scotoma is a visual field defect located between the blind spot and the macula. This location corresponds with the papillomacular nerve fiber layer bundle, which lies between the optic disc and the macula.

8. d. Proptosis, lid retraction, and lid lag are features of thyroid orbitopathy, which is not a medical emergency requiring immediate hospitalization. The other choices indicate features of (a) carotid dissection, (b) papilledema, and (c) CN III palsy with pupil involvement suggesting aneurysm, which are all considered medical emergencies.

9.   b.   A central scotoma with a temporal defect in the fellow eye is indicative of a junctional scotoma, which localizes to the anterior optic chiasm. All of the other choices can occur with a lesion of the posterior optic chiasm.

10.   b.   Visual cortex lesions, depending on their localization, are unique in their ability to cause temporal crescent sparing, foveal sparing, and a central homonymous hemianopia. However, involvement of the temporal crescent of the visual field can occur with lesions anywhere along the visual pathway and therefore does not localize to the occipital lobe.

11.   d.   Optic disc pallor can occur from the lateral geniculate nucleus forward, due to the fact that the ganglion cell axons synapse in the lateral geniculate. Therefore, lesions of the optic radiations or visual cortex will not cause optic disc pallor.

12.   d.   Optochoroidal shunt vessels occur on the optic disc in sphenoid wing meningioma, glaucoma, and papilledema but are not usually a characteristic of traumatic optic neuropathy. If these vessels were seen in a patient with trauma, the other conditions would need to be ruled out as well.

13.   c.   Optic disc hemorrhages are rare in optic neuritis, occurring in only about 6% of cases of papillitis. Optic disc hemorrhages are more common in the other choices.

14.   b.   The pattern of optic disc swelling follows the thickness of the neuroretinal rim. Therefore, the inferior and superior regions swell first, followed by nasal and then temporal regions of the optic disc. The temporal region of the disc would be the last to swell in papilledema but would be the region most likely to exhibit Paton's lines.

15.   d.   Hypoplastic discs could be unilateral or bilateral. If they are bilateral and profoundly hypoplastic, there is a greater chance of CNS or endocrine abnormalities.

16.   c.   Nonarteritic anterior ischemic optic neuropathy is not usually associated with pain. If there is pain, arteritic anterior ischemic optic neuropathy and GCA need to be considered. Optic neuritis classically presents with pain on eye movements, and an aneurysm is associated with head pain.

17. a. Pupil asymmetry is a factor of the efferent visual system, necessitating further evaluation into the parasympathetic and sympathetic systems. Anisocoria is not a feature of optic neuropathy. The pupil abnormality associated with optic neuropathy is a relative afferent pupillary defect, which can be present without anisocoria. The other choices do assess the optic nerve function.

18. a. Cataract does not cause an RAPD in the involved eye. If the cataract is dense, it may cause the appearance of a subtle RAPD in the fellow eye, because of significant light scattering in the involved eye.

19. a. Light-near dissociation can be caused by, among other things, a tonic pupil, tectal pupil, and aberrant regeneration of a CN III palsy. Although aberrant regeneration can occur with a compressive lesion of CN III, it never occurs with a CN III palsy from diabetes.

20. d. Anisocoria, with a greater difference in pupil size, indicates a problem with the parasympathetic system. An oculosympathetic paresis, or Horner syndrome, is a problem with the sympathetic system and therefore would have anisocoria with a greater difference in pupil size in dim illumination.

21. e. Horner syndrome is associated with a dilation lag, meaning that the anisocoria would be greater at 5 seconds than at 12 seconds into darkness.

22. c. MRI of the lumbar spine has no role in finding the etiology of a Horner syndrome, because the sympathetic pathway does not extend down to the lumbar spine but rather goes to the low cervical/high thoracic level before passing over the apex of the lung. The MRI/MRA may be needed to find a mass/carotid dissection. Neuroblastoma needs to be considered with a Horner syndrome in a child.

23. d. Heterochromia iridis does not definitely indicate a congenital Horner syndrome and is often present in other causes of childhood Horner syndrome. Therefore, especially in the setting of a recently noted ptosis, a work-up is necessary to rule out other causes, including a neuroblastoma.

24. d. A CN III palsy with features suggestive of an aneurysm is an emergent condition warranting immediate work-up and potential treatment of the aneurysm. Without treatment, the patient could die from a subarachnoid hemorrhage if the aneurysm ruptures.

25. d. Diplopia can occur with pseudotumor cerebri, as in any case of papilledema. However, in pseudotumor cerebri, the only neurologic deficit that can occur, as indicated by Dandy's modified criteria, is a CN VI palsy. The CN VI innervates only the lateral rectus. This muscle only acts to pull the eye out into abduction. Therefore, damage to this nerve would only cause a horizontal diplopia.

26. b. In a CN IV palsy, the superior oblique muscle is not fully functional and therefore cannot act to pull the eye downward or to intort the eye. This means that the problem eye is higher, with its image being the lower of the two images. Due to the fact that the eye will also be excyclotorted, this lower image will also be tilted.

27. e. Over 10 degrees of excyclotorsion is characteristic of a bilateral CN IV palsy, which often needs to be surgically corrected after waiting a year without resolution. The other choices are characteristic of bilateral CN IV palsies.

28. b. Because the patient has a left hyperdeviation, it would be a left CN IV palsy, which would have a greater left hypercomponent in right gaze and left head tilt. Because this is of recent onset, there would likely be not only objective excyclotorsion but also subjective excyclotorsion.

29. a. Slowed saccades (glissades) are a feature of a neurogenic (CN VI) etiology to the abduction deficit. With a restrictive process, the saccades would be of normal speed but would stop short due to the restrictive process.

30. d. The ocular effects of MG are ptosis and ocular motility defects. MG does not affect the pupils. It can be associated with a thymoma in about 10% of cases.

31. c. Although bilateral altitudinal defects can occur with NA-AION and retinal problems, another cause must be considered if the nerve and retina appear normal. The defects could represent a co-existent right inferior and left inferior homonymous hemianopia. Because the two parietal lobes have separate circulations, it would be unlikely for an infarct to affect both sides simultaneously. However, because the right and left occipital lobes can share a common circulation, they can both be affected at the same time from an infarct. Because the defects are inferior, this would mean the problem is above the calcarine fissure.

32. c. Oral prednisone alone, as shown in the ONTT, is contraindicated as an initial treatment for optic neuritis, due to its increased risk of recurrence of the optic neuritis. The treatment of choice for acute optic neuritis is IV methylprednisolone. MRI is warranted to assess the risk of developing associated MS. Other causes of optic neuritis, such as Lyme disease, must also be ruled out. If the patient is found to have MRI changes suggestive of a high risk of MS, immunomodulation therapy should be considered.

33. a. The optic neuritis treatment trial has shown that MRI is the best indicator of who will progress to MS.

34. b. Vertical nystagmus is indicative of a pathologic nystagmus and is not a feature of congenital nystagmus.

35. c. Due to the increased risk of bleeding, blood thinners are contraindicated in a hemorrhagic stroke. All of the other choices would potentially benefit from the use of antiplatelet and/or anticoagulant drugs.

36. c. Serum protein electrophoresis is not used in testing for myasthenia gravis. However, acetylcholine receptor antibodies are the blood test that is used to determine if the patient may have MG. This test is not positive on every patient with MG, especially ocular MG, and therefore a single-fiber EMG is often also needed to assess for characteristics of MG. A chest CT is used to look for a thymoma as an associated finding in MG in about 10% of patients.

37. b. Mestinon is used to block the enzyme from eliminating the acetylcholine in the neuromuscular junction. This would allow a greater concentration of acetylcholine to be available. This is a treatment for myasthenia gravis, which is a disorder affecting the acetylcholine receptors at the neuromuscular junction.

38. a. The inferior rectus muscle is the most commonly involved in thyroid orbitopathy, followed by the medial rectus.

39. b. Because of the infiltration of the muscle belly, the muscle becomes restrictive. Therefore, if the eye cannot move out, it is not because there is damage to the CN VI or weakness of the lateral rectus muscle but because the medial rectus is restricting the outward movement of the eye.

40.   c.   One-and-a-half syndrome occurs with a lesion of the CN VI
            nucleus and the MLF. The CN VI lesion causes a gaze palsy toward
            the side of the lesion. An MLF lesion causes an adduction deficit
            on the side of the lesion and an abducting nystagmus in the
            contralateral eye (an internuclear ophthalmoplegia). The name
            one-and-a-half syndrome is used because the patient cannot look
            to the right with both eyes and cannot look to the left with one eye.

Part 2 Recommended Reading

Books

Albert DM, Jakobiec FA: *Principles and practice of ophthalmology* (Vols 1-5), Philadelphia,
    2000, Saunders.

Arffa RC: *Grayson's diseases of the cornea,* ed 4, St Louis, 1998, Mosby.

Benjamin WJ, ed: *Borish's clinical refraction,* Philadelphia, 1998, Saunders.

Fingeret M, Lewis T: *Primary care of the glaucomas,* New York, 2000, McGraw-Hill.

Friedman N, Kaiser PK, Trattler W: *Review of ophthalmology,* Philadelphia, 2004, Saunders.

Higginbotham EJ, Lee DA, eds: *Clinical guide to glaucoma management,* Woburn, MA, 2004,
    Butterworth-Heinemann.

Kaiser PK, Friedman NJ, Pineda R: *The Massachusetts Eye and Ear Infirmary illustrated
    manual of ophthalmology,* ed 2, Philadelphia, 2004, Saunders.

Kanski JJ: *Clinical ophthalmology: a systematic approach,* ed 5, London, 2003, Elsevier,
    Health Sciences Division.

Kanski JJ: *Clinical ophthalmology: a test yourself atlas,* ed 2, London, 2002, Elsevier,
    Health Sciences Division.

Krachmer JH, Mannis MJ, Holland EJ: *Cornea,* ed 2, St Louis, 2004, Mosby.

Litwak AB: *Glaucoma handbook,* Boston, 2000, Butterworth-Heinemann.

Liu GT, Volpe NJ, Galetta SL: *Neuro-ophthalmology diagnosis and treatment,* Philadelphia,
    2001, Saunders.

Morrison, JC, Pollack IP: *Glaucoma science and practice,* New York, 2003, Thieme.

Remington LA: *Clinical anatomy of the visual system,* ed 2, London, 2004,
    Butterworth-Heinemann.

Roberts CM: *Quick consult to diagnosing and treating ocular disease,* Boston, 2002,
    Butterworth-Heinemann.

Spalton DJ, Hitchings RA, Hunte PA et al: *Atlas of clinical ophthalmology,* St Louis, 2004,
    Mosby.

Steinert RF: *Cataract surgery,* ed 2, Philadelphia, 2004, Saunders.

Miller NR, Newman NJ: *Walsh & Hoyt's clinical neuro-ophthalmology* (multivolume series),
    Baltimore, 1995, Williams & Wilkins.

Watson PG, et al: *The sclera and systemic disorders,* ed 2, Boston, 2004,
    Butterworth-Heinemann.

Internet

www.lib.uiowa.edu/hw/ophth/disease.html

www.revoptom.com/HANDBOOK/default.htm

Refractive, Oculomotor, Sensory, and Integrative Conditions

CHAPTER 26

Anomalies of Refraction: Ametropia

Nancy Peterson-Klein, James R. Miller,
Robert Buckingham, Michael P. Keating,
Bruce Morgan, Philip E. Walling

1. Keratometry readings are as follows:
    OD 42.75 @ 010; 44.00 @ 100
    OS 44.00 @ 170; 40.00 @ 080
    In what meridian would you position the axis of minus cylinder to correct the astigmatism?
    a. OD 100; OS 080
    b. OD 180; OS 090
    c. OD 010; OS 080
    d. OD 100; OS 170

2. The following procedures all attempt to relax or control the accommodative system when performing a subjective refraction except:
    a. cycloplegic refraction
    b. Jackson cross cylinder (JCC) testing
    c. overfogging procedures
    d. binocular refraction with the vectographic slide

3. A patient's distance refractive correction is +4.50 −3.00 × 040. If the examiner performs retinoscopy at 66²/₃ cm, what lens combination will be in the phoropter when a neutral reflex is observed in all meridians?
    a. +3.00 −3.00 × 040
    b. +6.00 −4.50 × 040
    c. +4.50 −3.00 × 040
    d. +6.00 −3.00 × 040

4. While scoping at a distance of 40 cm, you observe against motion in all meridians. A sphere lens of magnitude 4.00D makes the reflex neutral in all meridians. What should you record as your retinoscopy finding for the distance Rx?
    a. +1.50DS
    b. −6.50DS
    c. −1.50DS
    d. −6.00DS

5. Which of the following drugs does NOT induce some amount of cycloplegia?
    a. 2% homatropine
    b. 2.5% phenylephrine
    c. 1% cyclopentolate
    d. 1% tropicamide

6. While scoping at a distance of 66⅔ cm, you observe with motion in all meridians. A sphere lens of magnitude 1.00D makes the reflex neutral in all meridians. What should you record as your retinoscopy finding for the distance Rx?
    a. −2.50DS
    b. +1.00DS
    c. +2.50DS
    d. −0.50DS

7. What lens power is needed in the phoropter to obtain a neutral reflex on an unaccommodated emmetrope while scoping at 66⅔ cm?
    a. +1.00DS
    b. −1.50DS
    c. +1.50DS
    d. −2.50DS

8. While performing static retinoscopy at 50 cm using a plano mirror setting and a +2.00DS working lens, you observe "against" motion in both principal meridians, but the slower motion is in the vertical meridian. Which prescription is possible?
    a. −1.00 −2.00 × 090
    b. −2.00 −2.00 × 180
    c. +2.00 − 1.00 × 090
    d. +2.00 −2.00 × 180

9. The red markings on a JCC lens indicate the meridian:
    a. midway (45°) between the plus and minus power meridians
    b. of plus power, minus cylinder axis
    c. of plus power, plus cylinder axis
    d. of minus power, minus cylinder axis

10. Your patient's best visual acuity is achieved with $-3.00 -6.00 \times 095$.
    Her refractive error diagnosis for this eye would be classified as:
    a. a simple hyperopic astigmat, with-the-rule (WTR)
    b. a compound myopic astigmat, with-the-rule (WTR)
    c. a mixed astigmat, against-the-rule (ATR)
    d. a compound myopic astigmat, against-the-rule (ATR)

11. You are performing static retinoscopy at 50 cm with spheres only. You
    observe neutrality in the 180th meridian with a +1.00D lens and in the
    90th meridian with a +2.00D lens. What lens combination would
    correct the patient optimally at infinity according to this retinoscopy
    finding?
    a. plano -1.00×090
    b. plano -1.00×180
    c. $+1.00 -1.00 \times 090$
    d. $+1.00 -1.00 \times 180$

12. The Bichrome test assumes that when light is refracted by the
    human eye:
    a. the red portion of the spectrum will be refracted more than the
       green
    b. the green portion will be refracted more than the red
    c. the yellow portion will be refracted more than either the red
       or green
    d. the yellow portion will be refracted less than either the red
       or green

13. Your patient sees best in her right eye through $+3.00 -1.50 \times 175$.
    Assume she is viewing through her spherical equivalent lens power and
    you are testing for cylinder power at the correct axis. Which JCC lens
    choice will she prefer?
    a. $+0.50 -1.00 \times 085$
    b. $+0.50 -1.00 \times 175$
    c. $+0.50 -0.50 \times 175$
    d. $+0.50 -0.50 \times 085$

14. In the case of the uncorrected mixed astigmat:
    a. both line images are in front of the retina
    b. both line images are behind the retina
    c. one line image is behind the retina and one is in front of the
       retina
    d. one line image is in front of the retina and the other is on the retina

15. If a 32-year-old woman has keratometry readings OD of 41.00D @ 180; 44.62D @ 090, Javal's rule could predict an approximate astigmatic correction of
    a. −3.62 × 090
    b. −3.62 × 180
    c. −3.12 × 180
    d. −4.00 × 180

16. Net retinoscopy findings for an eye are −1.00 −1.00 × 180. With no lenses in place and the retinoscope mirror at plano, you should see:
    a. "with" motion in all meridians at a distance of 40 cm
    b. "against" motion in all meridians at a distance of 50 cm
    c. "against" motion in the vertical and "with" motion in the horizontal at 66⅔ cm
    d. both a and c are correct

17. If your patient reports the darkest line on a clock dial is 2-8, and the 1-7 and 3-9 are equally dark, you should set the minus cylinder axis at:
    a. 045 degrees
    b. 090 degrees
    c. 060 degrees
    d. 180 degrees

18. If the meridian of greatest curvature, i.e., highest dioptric power, on the cornea is the 79th meridian, we classify the patient's astigmatism as:
    a. against-the-rule
    b. with-the-rule
    c. symmetric
    d. asymmetric

19. You have determined the principal meridians using static retinoscopy and have neutralized one with sphere lenses. Now when you orient the streak parallel to the 125 meridian, you observe against motion. To neutralize this reflex, along which meridian should you align the minus cylinder axis?
    a. 080
    b. 035
    c. 125
    d. 170

20. Which two retinoscopic reflex characteristics are used to both determine the principal meridians and neutralize the reflex?
    a. brightness and speed
    b. speed and width
    c. skew and break
    d. brightness and width

21. A retinoscopist works at 66⅔ cm with a +1.50D working lens in place. At the start of retinoscopy, the examiner observes with motion in both principal meridians and the 090 meridian has the fastest with motion. What are the refractive diagnosis and type of astigmatism represented?
    a. CHA, ATR
    b. CHA, WTR
    c. MA, ATR
    d. SHA, WTR

22. When performing a prism dissociated blur balance procedure, which eye is associated with the top image?
    a. the eye with BO prism
    b. the eye with BD prism
    c. the eye with BI prism
    d. the eye with BU prism

23. When performing the binocular bichrome test, the desired end point is:
    a. red-green equal
    b. first red
    c. last red
    d. first green

24. Your retinoscopy finding in the right eye is −4.50 −1.25 × 170. What is the correct sequence for the JCC test?
    a. power check, axis check, power check
    b. axis check, power check
    c. power check, axis check
    d. axis check

25. After fogging and then finding the initial monocular best sphere OD, the following prescription was in the phoropter: −4.25 −1.25 × 165. This axis was correct via JCC but the cylinder power needed refinement by 0.75D more minus cylinder. What should have been the final prescription in the phoropter at the completion of JCC?
    a. −4.50 −2.00 × 165
    b. −4.25 −2.00 × 165
    c. −5.00 −1.25 × 165
    d. −4.00 −2.00 × 165

26. For a patient with best corrected visual acuities (VAs) of OD 20/15 and OS 20/30, which procedure would be appropriate?
    a. the prism dissociated bichrome balance test
    b. the alternate occlusion test
    c. the prism dissociated blur balance test
    d. all of the above are appropriate

27. For a patient with a prescription of OD −6.25DS and OS −3.75DS, which of the following diagnoses is most accurate?
    a. antimetropia
    b. pseudomyopia
    c. anisometropia
    d. amblyopia

28. After performing keratometry and astigmatic chart testing, you decide to set the correcting cylinder axis at 180 degrees in the phoropter. For this to be an accurate decision, which of the following must be true?
    a. the 090 meridian of the cornea was most steep
    b. the 6-12 o'clock spoke was most distinct
    c. the patient has with-the-rule astigmatism
    d. all of the above are true

29. What is the anticipated response from your patient during the binocular bichrome test when +0.25DS is added on top of the response that had elicited an "equal" response?
    a. the red side is clearer
    b. the red and green sides still appear equally clear
    c. the green side is clearer
    d. the red side is blurrier

30. To extend the range of the keratometer to evaluate a steep cornea:
    a. multiply the keratometry readings by a 0.85 conversion factor
    b. use a +1.25D trial lens
    c. multiply the keratometry readings by 1.50
    d. use a −1.00D trial lens

31. How much fogging is appropriate for performing the Jackson cross cylinder test?
    a. −1.50D
    b. +0.50D
    c. 0.00D
    d. +1.00D

32. The dioptric midpoint between the horizontal and vertical focal lines for an uncorrected astigmat is called the:
    a. conoid of Sturm
    b. circle of least confusion
    c. spherical equivalent
    d. blur ellipse

33. If a patient enters your office with a superficial foreign body in the left eye, you should take visual acuities of:
   a. the left eye only
   b. the right eye only
   c. both the right and left eyes
   d. do not attempt visual acuities until the foreign body is removed

34. Which of the following does NOT measure distance visual acuity?
   a. Kay picture test
   b. MacClure reading book
   c. Bailey Lovie No. 5 logMAR
   d. Keeler crowded and uncrowded cards

35. Which of the following distance visual acuity tests CANNOT be used with a mirrored system?
   a. Snellen acuity using a Bausch & Lomb projector
   b. vectographic slide using a Reichert projector
   c. Bailey Lovie No. 5 chart
   d. Cardiff acuity cards

36. The Cardiff visual acuity test is suitable for children from ages:
   a. 1 to 2 years
   b. 3 to 4 years
   c. 4 to 6 years
   d. 6 to 10 years

37. Which of the following visual acuity tests is NOT designed for children under 4 years old?
   a. Kay picture test
   b. Sheridan Gardiner test
   c. Snellen visual acuity test
   d. Cardiff visual acuity test

38. When performing Snellen visual acuity at a distance target, the patient cannot read the 20/400 line. What is the next step?
   a. stop visual acuity testing and record visual acuity as "worse than 20/400"
   b. perform visual acuity using the Feinbloom low vision chart
   c. perform count finger visual acuity testing
   d. walk the patient toward the chart

39. Which of the following automatic refractors has an open view to relax accommodation?
   a. Canon R-1
   b. Topcon RK-1
   c. Nidek AR-1000
   d. Grand Seiko WR-5100K

40. What would happen to the prescription if the patient were to accommodate excessively during the autorefraction?
   a. an increase in myopia
   b. an increase in hyperopia
   c. an increase in astigmatism
   d. there would be no change in the outcome

41. Instrument myopia is more common in:
   a. adults
   b. children
   c. myopic patients
   d. hyperopic patients

42. A subjective autorefractor allows the doctor to:
   a. test the patient's visual acuity
   b. adjust the results of the autorefractor
   c. test the patient for phoria measurements
   d. perform a refraction using the autorefractor

43. The instrument target in most autorefractors:
   a. is small to allow patients to relax their accommodation
   b. is always blurred to help with distance fixation
   c. requires the patient to fixate a moving object
   d. is meant to simulate distance fixation

44. The prescription in the right eye of a patient is plano -1.00×075. When the patient is not wearing glasses, what is the axis of the stenopaic slit that makes all distance objects clear?
   a. 015
   b. 075
   c. 105
   d. 165

45. The stenopaic slit is used:
   a. with a 20/40 Snellen target
   b. to find the amount of astigmatism
   c. to find the principal astigmatic meridian
   d. to determine the best axis for visual acuity

46. The stenopaic slits shown below are used to assess the prescription of
     an eye with astigmatism. When the stenopaic slit is held at position 1,
     the patient sees clearly with a +5.00D sphere, and when the stenopaic
     slit is held at position 2, the patient sees clearly with a –2.00D sphere.
     What is the patient's spectacle prescription?

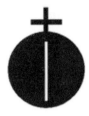 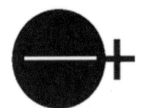

Position 1   Position 2

a. +5.00 –2.00 × 090
b. +5.00 –2.00 × 180
c. +5.00 –7.00 × 090
d. +5.00 –7.00 × 180

47. The stenopaic slits shown below are used to assess the prescription of
     an eye with astigmatism. When the stenopaic slit is held at position 1,
     the patient sees clearly with a –3.00D sphere, and when the stenopaic
     slit is held at position 2, the patient sees clearly with a –5.00D sphere.
     What is the patient's spectacle prescription?

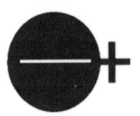 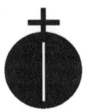

Position 1   Position 2

a. –2.00 –3.00 × 090
b. –3.00 –2.00 × 090
c. –3.00 –2.00 × 180
d. –5.00 –2.00 × 180

48. The stenopaic slit is similar in refractive properties to a:
     a. prism
     b. pinhole lens
     c. Maddox rod
     d. sunburst dial chart

49. The purpose of the Turville infinity balance is to:
    a. ensure each eye sees equally clear images
    b. ensure the refraction is equal between the two eyes
    c. equalize the best corrected visual acuity between the two eyes
    d. equalize the stimulus to accommodation between the two eyes

50. Which of the following IS NOT a step in the Turville infinity balance?
    a. separate the visual fields with a septum in the refracting lane
    b. fog both eyes with a +1.00D sphere
    c. allow each eye view of half of the chart
    d. insert prism before the two eyes

51. Which of the following problems would benefit from a Turville infinity balance?
    a. heterophoria
    b. latent nystagmus
    c. intermittent strabismus
    d. alternating heterotropia

52. The Turville infinity balance:
    a. allows the doctor to balance the eyes under binocular viewing conditions
    b. accounts for unequal object size differences
    c. presents the same image to both eyes
    d. is easy to set up

53. Which of the following is NOT true about the Turville infinity balance?
    a. allows for a natural viewing condition
    b. a septum is placed midway between the patient and the chart
    c. the right eye sees the left side of the chart and the left sees the other
    d. Turville infinity balance is based on the same idea as the bar reader

54. The purpose of the vectographic balance is to:
    a. check for suppression during the refraction
    b. allow fixation using both eyes simultaneously
    c. ensure the patient does not suppress the test letters
    d. ensure the stimulus for accommodation between the two eyes is equal

55. Another name for the "vectographic balance" is:
    a. filter technique
    b. Polaroid technique
    c. subjective polarization technique
    d. binocular balance without dissociation

56. Which of the following is NOT a step in the vectographic balance?
    a. place the Polaroid filters in front of both eyes
    b. fog both eyes with a +1.00D sphere
    c. allow each eye to view half of the chart
    d. prism dissociate the two eyes

57. The vectographic balance:
    a. allows the doctor to balance the eyes under monocular viewing conditions
    b. shows separate target simultaneously to the right and left eyes
    c. incorporates Polaroid filters to equalize image intensity
    d. presents the same image to both eyes

58. Which of the following is NOT true about the vectographic balance?
    a. is used on heterotropia patients
    b. allows for a normal viewing condition
    c. is the most natural binocular balance technique
    d. uses similar procedures as the vertical dissociation for balancing the eyes without the employment of prism

59. A 7-year-old girl with accommodative esotropia has a retinoscopy of +4.75DS in each eye without cycloplegia. If atropine were instilled, what would happen to the retinoscopy results?
    a. the cycloplegic retinoscopy would reveal more plus
    b. there would be no change in the refraction
    c. the pupils would dilate
    d. all of the above
    e. measure the refractive error in the absence of accommodation

60. The most common drug used in cycloplegic refractions is:
    a. atropine
    b. tropicamide
    c. homatropine
    d. cyclopentolate

61. Which of the following is NOT an indication for cycloplegic refraction?
    a. test for latent hyperopia
    b. assess the refractive status of children
    c. determine the refractive error in pre-presbyopia
    d. evaluate a patient with accommodative esotropia

62. Which of the following is the most important test that should be accomplished before a cycloplegic examination?
    a. measure the intraocular pressure in both eyes
    b. check the anterior chamber angles
    c. perform near point analysis
    d. accomplish frame selection

63. A 22-year-old man has accommodative esotropia, 0.7/0.8 cup-to-disc ratios, and has a retinoscopy of +5.25DS in each eye. Which of the following tests would be used to assist in the differential diagnosis of glaucoma?
    a. topography
    b. pachymetry
    c. keratometry
    d. subjective refraction

64. Which of the following patients would require a measurement of the corneal thickness?
    a. keratoconus patient
    b. LASIK surgery patient
    c. latent hyperopia patient
    d. irregular astigmatism patient

65. Which of the following is a normal corneal thickness?
    a. 373 microns
    b. 447 microns
    c. 556 microns
    d. 652 microns

Answers

1. c. The axis of minus cylinder correction should be placed coincident with the meridian of least corneal curvature to correct astigmatism.

2. b. Jackson cross cylinder testing refines the cylindrical component during a subjective refraction but does not relax or control accommodation.

3. d. The working distance adjustment for retinoscopy from $66^2/_3$ cm is −1.50D. Gross retinoscopic finding is +6.00 −3.00 × 040. The net retinoscopic finding is +4.50 −3.00 × 040.

4. b. Working distance adjustment for retinoscopy from 40 cm is −2.50D. The gross retinoscopic finding is −4.00DS. The net retinoscopic finding is −6.50DS.

5. b. Phenylephrine is a sympathomimetic and has no significant cycloplegic effect.

6. d. The working distance adjustment for retinoscopy from $66^2/_3$ cm is −1.50D. The gross retinoscopic finding is +1.00DS. The net retinoscopic finding is −0.50DS.

7. c. The working distance adjustment for retinoscopy from $66^2/_3$ cm is −1.50D. The gross retinoscopic finding is +1.50DS. The net retinoscopic finding is plano.

8. b. The working distance adjustment for retinoscopy from 50 cm is compensated for by the +2.00 working lens. Thus, against motion would put both image points in front of you and be considered compound myopic astigmatism. If the 090 meridian is slowest, it has more myopia than the 180 meridian resulting in WTR astigmatism. Only choice −2.00 −2.00 × 180 meets this criteria.

9. b. A cross cylinder lens has minus cylinder ground on one side and plus cylinder ground on the other with the two axes being 90 degrees apart. The red marking signifies the plus power and minus cylinder axis.

10. d. Both principal meridians are myopic, meeting the definition of compound myopic astigmatism, and the correcting cylinder axis is 090 or ATR.

11.   a.   Working distance adjustment for retinoscopy from 50 cm is −2.00D. Gross retinoscopic finding is +2.00 −1.00 × 090. Net retinoscopic finding is PL −1.00 × 090.

12.   b.   Green wavelengths of light are shorter and refracted less than the longer red wavelengths.

13.   b.   The spherical equivalent for +3.00 −1.50 × 175 is +2.25DS. Testing for cylinder power at the correct axis is 175. +0.50 −1.00 × 175 added to +2.25DS results in +2.75 −1.00 × 175 yielding the clearest lens choice.

14.   c.   A mixed astigmat has one myopic principal meridian resulting in a line image in front of the retina and one hyperopic principal meridian resulting in a line image behind the retina.

15.   d.   Javal's rule for estimated total astigmatism equals 1.25(ΔK) + (−0.50 × 090). ΔK = 44.62 − 41.00 = −3.62 × 180. 1.25 × −3.62 = −4.525 or −4.50 rounded to the nearest quarter diopter. −4.50 × 180 + −0.50 × 090 = −4.00 × 180.

16.   d.   Retinoscopy from 40 cm would have both image points behind you, 100 cm and 50 cm, and result in "with" motion in all meridians. Retinoscopy from 66²/₃ cm would have one image point behind you, 100 cm yielding "with" motion in the horizontal meridian and one image point in front of you, and 50 cm yielding "against" motion in the vertical meridian. Both a and c are correct.

17.   c.   Using the Rule of 30, take the smallest number on the darkest clock spoke and multiply by 30 to determine the appropriate axis of corrections: 2 × 30 = 60.

18.   b.   WTR astigmatism is defined as a cornea with the greatest meridian of curvature in the 90-degree meridian plus or minus 30 degrees.

19.   c.   With your streak oriented parallel to the 125 meridian, you are evaluating power in the 035 meridian. The minus cylinder axis must be placed at 125 to attempt to neutralize this against motion.

20.   d.   Brightness and width are the only two retinoscopic reflex characteristics used to both determine the principal meridians and neutralize the reflex.

21. b. Working distance adjustment for retinoscopy from 66⅔ cm is compensated for by the +1.50D working lens. Thus, with motion would put both image points behind you and be considered hyperopic or compound hyperopic astigmatism. If the 090 meridian is fastest, it has less hyperopia than the 180 meridian resulting in WTR astigmatism.

22. b. Base down prism moves the image up (top).

23. d. Fogging into the red and reducing the fog until first green discourages overminusing and is the desired end point.

24. b. When retinoscopy finds significant astigmatism, performing JCC should first refine the cylinder axis (axis check) and then refine the power (power check).

25. d. $-4.25 -1.25 \times 165$ was in the phoropter. After -0.50×165 was added, -0.25DS should be reduced to maintain the spherical equivalent yielding $-4.00 -1.75 \times 165$. Last, another -0.25×165 was added, resulting in $-4.00 -2.00 \times 165$.

26. a. A non–acuity-based test is indicated for patients with unequal acuities. The prism dissociated bichrome balance test is not acuity based.

27. c. Unequal refractive error between two eyes is diagnosed as anisometropia.

28. d. The correcting cylinder axis set at 180 degrees corrects for WTR astigmatism, which by definition is most steep in the 90 meridian and by using the Rule of 30 in reverse would report the 6-12 spoke as most distinct. All are true.

29. a. An equal response on the Bichrome test places the patient in the center of the chromatic interval with the green in front of the retina and the red behind. Adding +0.25DS shifts the intervals into the vitreous, making the red side appear clearer.

30. b. A +1.25DS trial lens taped over the end of the keratometer with the flattest side facing the eyepiece extends the range for steeper measurements.

31. c. Jackson cross cylinder testing is not performed under fogged conditions.

32. b. The circle of least confusion is at the dioptric midpoint of the conoid of Sturm.

33. c. The visual acuity of both eyes should be attempted prior to removal of any foreign body.

34. b. The MacClure reading book is a near visual acuity test.

35. c. Bailey Lovie cards should not be used through a mirrored system and should be tested directly at 6 M.

36. a. The Cardiff visual acuity test is suitable for children aged 1 to 2 years.

37. c. The Snellen visual acuity test may be too advanced for a 4-year-old patient.

38. d. When the patient is unable to read the 20/400 letter, the next step is to have the patient walk toward the chart to check if he is able to read the 20/400 letter at a closer distance.

39. d. The Grand Seiko WR-5100K has an open view to allow patients an unrestricted binocular view of a natural distance target.

40. a. As a patient accommodates, the prescription becomes more myopic.

41. b. Children have a tendency to accommodate during the measurement process.

42. d. Perform a subjective refraction using the autorefractor.

43. d. The instrument target is meant to simulate distance fixation.

44. b. For a stenopaic slit, the axis of the slit will be the axis of the prescription.

45. c. The primary use of the stenopaic slit is to locate the principal astigmatic meridian.

46. d. +5.00 −7.00 × 180; the axis is 90 degrees from the power of the cylinder. The difference between the two meridians is −7.00 D.

47. b. −3.00 −2.00 × 090

48. b. The stenopaic slit is an elongated pinhole.

49. d. Equalize the stimulus for accommodation between the two eyes.

50. d. Prism dissociation is not a technique used in the Turville infinity balance.

51. b. Patients with latent nystagmus will not exhibit the nystagmus movement because of the peripheral fusion lock.

52. a. The Turville infinity balance allows the doctor to perform a balance under binocular viewing conditions.

53. c. The right eye sees the right side of the chart, and the left sees the left side of the chart.

54. d. The primary purpose of all balance tests is to equalize the stimulus for accommodation between the two eyes.

55. b. The vectographic balance uses a Polaroid lens, allowing each eye to view separate but similar images.

56. d. Prism dissociation is not a technique used in the vectographic balance.

57. b. The vectographic balance shows separate targets simultaneously to both eyes under binocular conditions.

58. a. Vectographic balance cannot be used on heterotropia patients.

59. a. Atropine will reveal more plus on an accommodative esotropia patient.

60. c. Most doctors use cyclopentolate when performing a cycloplegic refraction.

61. c. Cycloplegic refractions are indicated in testing for latent hyperopia, assessing the refraction in children, and evaluating accommodative esotropia.

62. b. The doctor must check the anterior chamber angles to rule out the risk of angle closure.

63. b. Pachymetry should be performed to evaluate the thickness of the cornea.

64. b. Even though you may want to measure corneal thickness on a keratoconus patient, a LASIK surgery patient must have pachymetry before the surgery.

65. c. Below 500 microns is considered thin, and above 600 microns is considered thick.

CHAPTER 27

Anomalies of Refraction: Presbyopia

Nancy Peterson-Klein, James R. Miller,
Robert Buckingham, Michael P. Keating,
Bruce Morgan, Philip E. Walling

1. Presbyopia is clinically defined as a reduction in accommodative amplitude in a patient with a proper distance correction who can no longer perform near tasks at a customary working distance without experiencing near symptoms. The onset of presbyopia depends on:
   a. habitual working and reading distances
   b. lag of accommodation
   c. size of the pupil
   d. environmental temperature changes

2. Add values for the correction of presbyopia can be based on age. What add power would you expect to prescribe as a tentative add for a 50-year-old patient using Hofstetter's rule (average) and keeping one half of the amplitude in reserve?
   a. 0.75
   b. 1.00
   c. 1.25
   d. 1.50

3. What solution or solutions do patients resort to using to see clearly at the near point as the amplitude of accommodation decreases to the point that the patient cannot see clearly at near point?
   a. allow the print to blur slightly and take advantage of the depth of focus
   b. increase the reading distance by holding the work farther from the eye
   c. use all of the amplitude despite the large effort required to obtain the last portion of the amplitude
   d. avoid the problem by decreasing the amount of near work
   e. all of the above

4. The cross cylinder method used for the determination of the tentative addition creates artificial astigmatism. When the circle of least confusion is focused on the retina by spherical lenses with the cross cylinder positioned with minus axis vertical, the patient:
   a. will report the vertical lines darker or blacker
   b. will report the horizontal lines darker or blacker
   c. will not see the lines
   d. will report the vertical and horizontal lines as being equally distinct

5. The technique called "plus buildup," used for the determination of the tentative addition, uses plus powered lenses in 0.25D increments over the final distance correction until reaching the appropriate end point. The tentative add would represent the:
   a. difference between distance correction and final near correction that provided first blur of the 20/30 letters
   b. difference between distance correction and final near correction that provided least amount of plus to read 20/30 letters clearly
   c. difference between distance correction and final near correction that provided half a diopter more plus power (or less minus power) to read 20/30 letters clearly
   d. none of the above

6. With a declining amplitude of accommodation and an increasing near addition, the near point of accommodation through the distance portion moves farther from the patient, and the far point of accommodation through the near portion moves closer to the patient. When a physical range of blurred vision exists between the near point of accommodation through the distance portion and the far point of accommodation through the near portion, the patient is a candidate for a trifocal. This range begins when the near addition is:
   a. +1.25D
   b. +1.50D
   c. +1.75D
   d. +2.50D

7. It is generally accepted that the clinician should keep the presbyopic addition power as weak as possible because:
   a. the patient loses his or her accommodative ability faster with higher adds
   b. lower adds create the deepest range of clear vision
   c. the adaptation occurs slower with lower addition powers
   d. none of the above

8. The habitual Rx is +4.00 – 2.00 × 90 with a +1.50D add. The distance subjective refraction revealed +4.50 –2.00 × 90. The tentative add determination revealed a +1.75D add. How would you write the prescription if the patient desired an updated single vision reading prescription (Rx)?
   a. +2.50 –2.00 × 90
   b. +1.75 –2.00 × 90
   c. +6.25 –2.00 × 90
   d. +4.50 –2.00 × 90

9. The results of accommodative facility testing for a 38-year-old patient are as follows: OU 6 cpm (decay with minus), OD 6 cpm (decay with minus), OS 7 cpm (decay with minus). What is the likely diagnosis?
   a. convergence excess
   b. pre-presbyopia
   c. convergence insufficiency
   d. basic eso

10. A 46-year-old patient has never worn glasses and has no symptoms. The subjective refraction is OD: plano and OS: –1.50DS. Accommodative amplitude is 4.50D and the fused-X cylinder test results yield +1.50D, with 20/20 in each eye at 40 cm. What prescription would you recommend?
    a. no prescription
    b. distance only
    c. bifocal
    d. trifocal

11. What are the most common causes of unequal adds?
    a. inaccurate distance refraction
    b. unilateral pseudophakia
    c. unilateral aphakia corrected by a contact lens
    d. unilateral accommodative palsy
    e. all of the above

12. Two bifocal side effects are image jump and optical displacement. The optical jump is due to:
    a. the power of the distance correction and the distance of the dividing line from the optical center of the segment
    b. the power of the add and the distance of the dividing line from the optical center of the segment
    c. the prismatic effects of the distance correction
    d. none of the above

13. It is important to consider all the diverse visual needs of adult presbyopic patients. One standard "pearl of prescribing" is to:
    a. measure the segment height with the patient's head in its natural position when looking straight ahead (be sure to be on the same eye level with patient)
    b. never recommend multiple prescriptions for different tasks (most patients only want one pair of glasses to fit all needs)
    c. change segment height to the correct level if the bifocal is too low, even though the patient is happy with the habitual segment height
    d. convince patients of the value of progressives because that lens design is better cosmetically than segment bifocals

14. The patient has a distance Rx of −1.25D OU with a +1.25D add. The patient does not want a bifocal or PAL but desires one pair of spectacles for distance and another for near. What power would you prescribe for near use?
    a. −1.25D
    b. +2.50D
    c. plano
    d. +1.25D

15. What power would you measure in the bifocal add portion of the Rx with the lensometer if the distance Rx is −5.00D and the add is +1.50D?
    a. +1.50D
    b. −3.50D
    c. −6.50D
    d. none of the above

16. Your patient has an Rx of −3.00D with a +2.50D add and is corrected with contact lenses for distance with an overrefraction of plano. He wants glasses for computer use only. You determine a +1.75D add is best for computer use. What Rx should the patient wear over his contact lenses for computer use?
    a. +1.75D
    b. +2.50D
    c. −0.50D
    d. +1.25D

17. For the patient in Question #16, what single vision spectacle Rx would you give him to wear for his computer work when he is not wearing his contact lenses?
    a. +1.75D
    b. −0.50D
    c. −1.25D
    d. +2.50D

18. You examine a patient in a "short room" and find the following Rx, distance +2.25DS with a +2.00D add. You decide to reduce the distant Rx by 0.25D (or 0.25D more − or less +) to allow for the short room. What add will you give?
    a. +1.75D
    b. +4.00D
    c. +2.00D
    d. +2.25D

19. A patient has a distance Rx of −2.00DS. You need to perform a visual field using a Humphrey field analyzer. The recommended add to use is +3.00D. What lens do you place in the lens holder of the instrument?
    a. +1.00D
    b. +2.00D
    c. +3.00D
    d. −1.00D

20. Monovision is the technique of fitting contact lenses so that one eye is corrected for distance and the other eye is corrected for near. If a patient has a spectacle Rx for distance of OD −3.00DS, OS −2.50DS with a +2.50D add, and you were to fit the right eye for distance and the left eye for near, what powers would you need?
    a. OD −0.50D, OS no lens
    b. OD −3.00D, OS +2.50D
    c. OD no lens, OS +2.50D
    d. OD −3.00D, OS no lens

21. Which of the following prescriptions represent a significant increase in the total net plus power at near?
    a. OU: +2.00DS/+2.00D add
    b. OU: +3.00DS/+1.00D add
    c. OU: +3.00DS/+2.00D add
    d. OU: +3.00DS/+1.50D add

22. What epidemiological factors do not have any effects on the development of presbyopia?
    a. age
    b. nutritional factors
    c. average annual temperature
    d. exposure to ultraviolet radiation
    e. none of the above

Answers

1. a. Patients are unaware of near blur if they hold their reading task farther away than normal reading distances. As a general rule, reading near print will be comfortable if one half the amplitude of accommodation is kept in reserve. When reading distances violate that rule, then the onset of presbyopia results.

2. c. Hofstetter's formula (average): 18.5 − 0.3 (age) equals the average amplitude for the age. 18.5 − 0.3 (50) = 2.50. Tentative add = 1.25, to keep one half the amplitude in reserve.

3. e. Strategies b and d are often used, but the patient may use each strategy at different times.

4. d. Accommodation or adequate spherical lenses move the interval of Sturm so the circle of least confusion in the astigmatic interval is on the retina. If the horizontal lines are reported blacker, then the interval is positioned farther behind the retina, and vice versa if the vertical lines are blacker.

5. b. Higher adds than necessary affect the patient's customary near visual habits, mostly the decrease in the far point through the correction. The higher add also reduces the range of clear vision. Prescribe the least plus power in order for the patient to read the letters clearly.

6. c. Before writing a prescription, the clinician should demonstrate the range of clear vision through the tentative distance and near corrections to show the patient this range or gap of indistinct vision and how the intermediate distance can be cleared with a trifocal.

7. b. Higher adds affect the patient's customary near visual habits, mostly the decrease in the far point of accommodation through the correction.

8. c. Combine the distance sphere power with the near reading tentative add along with the distance cylindrical power and axis. +4.50 −2.00 × 90 + (+1.75DS) = +6.25 −2.00 × 90.

9. b. An older patient who is presbyopic or pre-presbyopic may show a low-facility measurement because of the inability to accommodate enough to see through the minus side of the flippers. (If the target is held at 40 cm [2.50D] and −2.00D lenses are used in the flipper, the patient needs at least 4.50D of accommodation to clear the target.)

10. a. Providing an Rx for driving would blur the dashboard and require removal of glasses to view printed directions. A multifocal would restrict the near field of view compared to her uncorrected abilities. The effective add of +1.50D that she has by not correcting the −1.50D prescription in the eye is sufficient for her current accommodative demand. Do not try to improve an asymptomatic state.

11. d. Myopia OU reduced from previous correction. Confirm these findings with trial lenses. This reduction provides more "plus" power at near and improves clarity of fine print.

12. b. Image jump results from the difference in prismatic effects between distance and reading portions at their junction. Review Prentice's rule.

13. a. Parallax from unequal positions of patient and designer/fitter cause the seg height to be too high or too low.

14. c. Reading Rx equals the algebraic result of the distance correction and the addition power. −1.25 + (+1.25) = plano or zero. The clinical answer is for the patient to remove the distance Rx for reading tasks.

15. b. Reading Rx equals the algebraic result of the distance correction and the addition power.

16. a. The plano overrefraction indicates the contact lens power has been compensated in power to correct for the vertex distance. The proper add would be +1.75D for use over the contact lenses.

17. c. −3.00 + (+1.75) = −1.25 to obtain the single vision computer Rx. The uncorrected −1.75DS serves as the "built-in" add for computer viewing.

18. d. Compensate for the reduced + power at distance by increasing the add power by +0.25D so the total net power at near does not change.

19. a. Use the concept of the "built-in" add of uncorrected myopia of −2.00D and combine with a +1.00D trial lens to obtain +3.00D testing distance "lens."

20. e. Correct the distance eye with −3.00D and prescribe no lens in the other eye due to the "built-in" near addition.

21. c. Combine the distance correction with the near add to obtain the total net correction for reading: +3.00 + (+2.00) = +5.00DS net correction for reading.

22. e. Poor nutrition disrupts normal metabolic function of the crystalline lens. Age has represented the most tangible indication that a patient is likely to be presbyopic. Populations with close proximity to equator and with higher temperatures have shown presbyopic onset at earlier ages than do European populations.

CHAPTER 28

Anomalies of Refraction: Aphakia, Pseudophakia, and Aniseikonia

Nancy Peterson-Klein, James R. Miller, Robert Buckingham, Michael P. Keating, Bruce Morgan, Philip E. Walling

1. Aniseikonia is a _____ condition where retinal _____ differ in size.
   a. binocular, objects
   b. binocular, images
   c. monocular, objects
   d. monocular, images

2. The perceived image size difference due to unequal prism effects when viewing through different parts of two anisometropic spectacle lenses is known as:
   a. spectacle aniseikonia
   b. dynamic aniseikonia
   c. induced aniseikonia
   d. phoric aniseikonia

3. The two most common clinical symptoms of aniseikonia are:
   a. headache and asthenopia
   b. distortion and anisometropia
   c. distortion and reading difficulty
   d. photophobia and anisometropia

4. In general, a person with aphakic spectacles will have _____ compared with a person with pseudophakic spectacles.
   a. a decreased convergence demand and an increased barrel distortion
   b. an increased convergence demand and an increased barrel distortion
   c. an increased convergence demand and an increased pincushion distortion
   d. a decreased convergence demand and an increased pincushion distortion

5. The two methods of measuring aniseikonia are:
   a. direct comparison and space perception
   b. direct evaluation and indirect comparison
   c. space alteration and space reorganization
   d. direct evaluation and anisometropia comparison

6. All of the following can be used to test for aniseikonia EXCEPT:
   a. eikonometer
   b. aniseikonia inspector
   c. aniseikonia evaluator
   d. new aniseikonia test

7. A patient with OD +5.00 −5.00 × 180 and OS +5.00 −5.00 × 090 has meridional aniseikonia. Meridional aniseikonia produces:
   a. differences in target size
   b. meridional anisometropia
   c. distorted space perception
   d. lateral and vertical heterophoria

8. A 24-year-old monocular pseudophakic patient has a spectacle prescription of OD +9.00DS and OS plano −0.50 × 090. Which is the least important when considering the management of the patient's spectacles?
   a. lens material
   b. frame material
   c. size of the frame
   d. aspheric lens design

9. A 34-year-old binocular pseudophakic patient has a spectacle prescription of OD +8.00 −2.50 × 180 and OS −0.50 −3.50 × 180. The doctor decides to correct the anisometropia with contact lenses. What else should the doctor prescribe?
   a. sunglasses
   b. artificial tears
   c. reading glasses
   d. tinted contact lenses

10. The two main causes of anomalous aniseikonia are differences in:
   a. retinal image size and photoreceptor spacing
   b. spectacle prescriptions and corneal curvature
   c. corneal curvature and lateral heterophoria
   d. object size and spectacle prescriptions

11. The clinical rule of thumb for aniseikonia management is that for
   every 1.00D of anisometropia, there is a _____ aniseikonia.
   a. 0.5%
   b. 1.0%
   c. 1.5%
   d. 2.0%

12. All of the following are clinical reasons for anatomical aniseikonia
   EXCEPT:
   a. central serous chorioretinopathy
   b. open angle glaucoma
   c. epiretinal membrane
   d. scleral buckle

13. When altering the magnification in aphakic spectacles, which of the
   following parameters is the *least* acceptable to change?
   a. power
   b. base curve
   c. refractive index
   d. center thickness

14. In general, an aphakic patient with a +15.00DS OU will be prescribed
   what type of lenses for their spectacles?
   a. Varilux lenses
   b. myodisc lenses
   c. iseikonic lenses
   d. lenticular lenses

15. All of the following objective tests should be included in the
   management of a pseudophakic patient EXCEPT:
   a. biomicroscopy
   b. chief complaint
   c. refraction examination
   d. binocular indirect ophthalmoscopy

16. All of the following are inherent disadvantages of wearing aphakic
   spectacles EXCEPT:
   a. weight of the glasses
   b. excessive temple length
   c. "jack in the box" ring scotoma
   d. cosmetically the eye appears unusually large

17. A 65-year-old woman has cataracts and decides to have cataract surgery with an intraocular lens implant. During the operation, the surgeon ruptures the posterior capsule. Without getting a different lens, the surgeon decides to place the lens in the sulcus instead of the capsular bag. What would happen to the postoperative refraction from what you would have anticipated?
    a. the patient is more myopic
    b. the patient is more hyperopic
    c. the patient is more presbyopic
    d. no change; the patient has the same refraction as what you would anticipate preoperatively

18. Which option is the best option to correct for unilateral aphakia in a pediatric patient?
    a. IOL
    b. LASIK
    c. spectacles
    d. contact lens

Answers

1. b. Aniseikonia is a binocular phenomenon in which the retinal images are of different size.

2. b. Dynamic aniseikonia is aniseikonia caused by the prismatic effect of looking through the peripheral portions of anisometropic lenses.

3. a. The most common clinical symptoms of aniseikonia are headache and asthenopia.

4. c. Due to the large plus power of aphakic spectacles, the person will notice an increased convergence demand and increased pincushion distortion compared with normal spectacles.

5. a. There are two methods of measuring aniseikonia. Direct comparison uses different size targets presented to the patient, while space perception uses a space eikonometer.

6. c. There is no aniseikonia evaluator test. The three tests are the eikonometer, aniseikonia inspector, and the new aniseikonia test.

7. c. Meridional aniseikonia produces distorted space perception rather than image size differences.

8. b. Lens material, lens design, and frame size are very important to reduce the weight of the lenses. Frame material is the least important.

9. c. Sunglasses, artificial tears, and tinted contact lenses are options. However, because the patient has binocular pseudophakia, he or she will not be able to read. Reading glasses over the contact lenses should be prescribed.

10. a. Aniseikonia is caused from differences in retinal image size. This can be caused by difference between the two eyes in spacing of the photoreceptors.

11. b. The general rule is that for every 1.0D of difference between the power of the anisometropia, there will be a corresponding 1% aniseikonia.

12. b. Anatomical aniseikonia can be caused by any disease that will elongate or shorten the eye causing an anisometropia. Open angle glaucoma will not elongate or shorten the eye compared with an epiretinal membrane, central serous chorioretinopathy, and scleral buckle.

13. a. If the doctor changes the power of a spectacle prescription, the patient's vision may become blurred. To decrease the magnification, the doctor should change the base curve, index of refraction, and center thickness.

14. d. Lenticular lenses are used for patients with large plus prescriptions.

15. b. The chief complaint is not an objective test; it is a subjective response from the patient.

16. b. Aphakic spectacles produce excessive weight and a "jack in the box" ring scotoma, and the eye appears unusually large. Excessive temple length is not an inherent problem with aphakic spectacles.

17. a. By placing the lens in the sulcus, the focal point is moved anteriorly and the patient becomes myopic. Ideally, if the lens were to be placed in the sulcus, the power of the lens should be reduced by about 0.50D from that calculated preoperatively. Normally, surgeons will have multiple lenses available at the time of surgery to avoid this problem.

18. d. For unilateral aphakia, an extended wear, high oxygen–permeable contact lens is the method of choice for correcting the aphakia.

CHAPTER **29**

Low Vision

Lewis Reich, Dawn DeCarlo

CONTENT AREAS

- Epidemiology and history
- Clinical signs, techniques, and skills for determining a correction
  - Visual acuity
  - Special refraction techniques
  - Visual fields
  - Reading skills
  - Effects of illumination
  - Magnification determination
  - In-office evaluation with low vision devices
- Diagnosis and treatment
- Management and prognosis
  - Analysis and interpretation of personal, social, vocational, and psychological patient needs and factors
  - Prescribing low vision devices with reference to magnification, full field of view, and working distance
  - Patient education and training
  - Roles and relationships with other disciplines
  - Prognostic factors and follow-up care

1. What is the leading cause of vision impairment in adults over age 80?
   a. glaucoma
   b. cataract
   c. diabetic retinopathy
   d. age-related macular degeneration

2. Which of the following problems would least likely be reported by a patient with age-related macular degeneration presenting for low vision evaluation?
   a. bumping into walls
   b. poor performance in dim illumination
   c. difficulty reading the newspaper
   d. inability to recognize faces

3. The most common inherited eye disease associated with vision impairment is:
   a. retinitis pigmentosa
   b. albinism
   c. rod monochromatism (achromatopsia)
   d. Stargardt's macular degeneration
   e. Leber's hereditary optic neuropathy

4. Which of the following conditions is LEAST likely to lead to total blindness?
   a. retinitis pigmentosa
   b. diabetic retinopathy
   c. glaucoma
   d. hereditary optic atrophy

231

5. Professionals other than optometrists who may be involved in the rehabilitative process of visually impaired individuals include all of the following EXCEPT:
    a. psychologists
    b. social workers
    c. occupational therapists
    d. teachers
    e. a, b, c, and d

6. Functionally, the most difficult position for reading with eccentric viewing is:
    a. 12 o'clock
    b. 3 o'clock
    c. 6 o'clock
    d. 9 o'clock

7. A monocular patient with a −5.00 DS OD uncorrected refractive error is using a +14-D microscope OD. How far from the lens should you instruct them to hold their reading material?
    a. 3.6 inches
    b. 5.2 inches
    c. 2.0 inches
    d. 9.0 inches

8. A manufacturer wishes to label a +10-D hand-held magnifier based on a 40-cm reference distance. The magnification would be:
    a. ×2.5
    b. ×3.5
    c. ×4
    d. ×5

9. A Keplerian telescope that is labeled as having ×4 magnification is adjusted in length to focus an object that is 25 cm in front of its +20-D objective lens. The equivalent power is:
    a. +12 D
    b. +16 D
    c. +20 D
    d. +80 D

10. A patient's best-corrected near acuity is 0.25/16 M. She wants to read the newspaper (1 M) with the CCTV while sitting 40 cm away from the monitor. How tall should the letters be on the screen?
    a. 23.20 mm
    b. 37.12 mm
    c. 14.50 mm
    d. 6.89 mm

11. A patient uses a flexible arm lamp for reading. If the lamp is moved from 50 cm to 25 cm from the reading material, what is the effect on the illumination?
    a. ×1, no change
    b. ×2
    c. ×4
    d. ×0.25

12. A patient is able to clearly see a distant target while looking through an afocal ×3.0 telescope when a +0.5-D lens is held over the objective lens. The approximate refractive error of this patient is closest to:
    a. +0.50 D
    b. +3.00 D
    c. +4.50 D
    d. +9.00 D

13. A patient presents with 20/120 distance visual acuity. What power hand-held Jackson cross cylinder would be MOST appropriate to use based upon the principle of just noticeable difference (JND)?
    a. ±0.25 D
    b. ± 0.50 D
    c. ± 0.75 D
    d. ±1.00 D

14. Which of the following lens designs should be avoided to minimize distortions when used as a high-power spectacle-mounted magnifying system?
    a. spherical biconvex
    b. aplanatic doublet
    c. achromatic doublet
    d. aspheric

15. A 70-year-old patient with macular degeneration has 20/30 visual acuity, yet presents with multiple visual complaints including severe difficulty identifying faces. Which of the following ancillary tests would be MOST appropriate?
    a. color vision
    b. electroretinography
    c. contrast sensitivity
    d. 30-2 threshold Humphrey visual field

16. Which of the following patients would be MOST likely to present with symptoms of depression?
    a. patient with new-onset unilateral visual acuity loss
    b. patient with recent-onset bilateral visual acuity loss
    c. patient with longstanding bilateral visual acuity loss
    d. patient with longstanding bilateral visual field loss

17. Which of the following telescopes would provide the dimmest image of an extended object for a patient with a 4-mm pupil?
    a. 4×16
    b. 4×20
    c. 4×12
    d. 4×8

18. A 60-year-old emmetropic low vision patient can use a +8-D hand-held magnifier for reading her pill bottle. For some reason, she insists on using this hand-held magnifier while viewing through her +4-D single vision reading glasses. How far away from the spectacle plane must the hand-held magnifier be held so she has a total equivalent power of +8.0 D?
    a. 12.5 cm
    b. 25 cm
    c. 8.3 cm
    d. 40 cm

19. Which of the following would decrease the field of view for a patient using a hand-held magnifier?
    a. increase lens diameter of the hand-held magnifier
    b. increase distance between hand-held magnifier and the eye
    c. decrease the power of the lens in the hand-held magnifier
    d. decrease the index of refraction of lens

20. A Galilean telescope has a 15-mm entrance pupil and a 5-mm exit pupil. This telescope would accurately be labeled:
    a. 5×15
    b. 3×15
    c. 3×5
    d. 5×3

21. Due to physical limitations, a presbyopic low vision patient is unable to maintain a stable working distance for reading tasks. Which of the following devices would be most successful for this patient?
    a. CCTV
    b. spectacle microscope
    c. hand-held magnifier
    d. telemicroscope

22. Your low vision patient likes to watch television in the evenings. However, he reports significant difficulties in following his programs because he is unable to clearly view the screen. Which would be the LEAST beneficial management option?
    a. Fresnel-type TV magnifier
    b. increase in the size of the screen
    c. decrease the viewing distance
    d. close focus telescope or telemicroscope

23. In many states, low vision patients can drive using bioptic telescopes that are mounted in a spectacle carrier lens containing the prescription (if any is required). What is the most correct division of time that a properly trained driver will spend viewing through the telescope and through the spectacle carrier lens?
     a. 95% through the telescope, 5% through the spectacle carrier
     b. 70% through the telescope, 30% through the spectacle carrier
     c. 50% through the telescope, 50% through the spectacle carrier
     d. 5% through the telescope, 95% through the spectacle carrier

24. A patient reads 0.4/4-M single letters using the appropriate add. Which telemicroscope would permit her to just resolve 1-M letters?
     a. ×1.5 telescope with +6-D reading cap
     b. ×2 telescope with +4-D reading cap
     c. ×3 telescope with +3-D reading cap
     d. ×4 telescope with +2.5-D reading cap

25. The emotional response to permanent visual loss has been characterized by five distinct stages. The initial stage is:
     a. denial
     b. anger
     c. bargaining
     d. depression

26. You have a patient who has previously been diagnosed with oculocutaneous albinism. Assume that there are no other ocular abnormalities. When performing testing as part of your low vision evaluation, you may find all of the following EXCEPT:
     a. photophobia
     b. color vision abnormalities
     c. reduced visual acuity
     d. nystagmus

27. A patient with which of the following diagnoses has the best potential for being a safe driver assuming that the patient also has 20/70 distance visual acuity and long-standing disease duration?
     a. diabetic retinopathy with a history of panretinal photocoagulation
     b. primary open angle glaucoma
     c. retinitis pigmentosa
     d. macular hole

28. A stand magnifier is constructed such that the +15-D lens is 5 cm above the reading text. What is the maximum add power that can be used to view the image created by this stand magnifier?
    a. 4 D
    b. 5 D
    c. 10 D
    d. 2.5 D

29. When treating a patient with Fresnel prisms, how should the prism be oriented for visual field enhancement in a patient with a left homonymous hemianopsia?
    a. base-in OS over the nasal portion of the lens
    b. base-in OS over the temporal portion of the lens
    c. base-out OS over the nasal portion of the lens
    d. base-out OS over the temporal portion of the lens

30. A patient with age-related macular degeneration has developed subretinal neovascularization that ultimately has caused his visual acuity to drop by 0.6 logMAR. If his initial visual acuity was measured to be 20/50, what is his new visual acuity?
    a. 20/50
    b. 20/80
    c. 20/100
    d. 20/200

Answers

1. d. Prevalence data on eye disease in the United States published in
        Archives of Ophthalmology (volume 122, April 2004) indicate that
        11.8% of Americans over age 80 have advanced age-related macular
        degeneration (ARMD) and 23.6% have intermediate ARMD,
        compared with 7.7% with glaucoma. Diabetic retinopathy affects
        5.8% of those over age 75. Cataract is a highly prevalent yet
        treatable condition that rarely leads to vision impairment.

2. a. Macular degeneration is a disease whose hallmark feature is
        decreased central visual acuity, making facial recognition and
        reading difficult. Patients with macular degeneration tend to perform
        much better in conditions of bright illumination and often require
        task lighting. Peripheral vision is well maintained, and therefore
        mobility is usually not a problem.

3. a. Fifteen percent of hereditary blindness is due to retinitis pigmentosa
        (RP). While albinism and Stargardt's macular degeneration are less
        common than RP, they are not as rare as rod monochromatism or
        Leber's hereditary optic neuropathy.

4. d. Retinitis pigmentosa can lead to complete blindness through
        photoreceptor apoptosis. Diabetic retinopathy can cause total
        blindness if neovascularization leads to tractional retinal detachment
        or anterior segment neovascularization and subsequent secondary
        neovascular glaucoma. Glaucoma can cause complete atrophy of the
        optic nerve and blindness. Hereditary optic atrophy primarily affects
        the temporal optic nerve with an average final acuity of 20/200 or
        better.

5. e. Optometric low vision rehabilitation consists largely of prescription
        of glasses and optical devices as well as training. All of the above
        professionals can be instrumental in the rehabilitation of the patient
        with low vision.

6. b. Three o'clock is the most difficult eccentric viewing position for
        reading (for all languages reading left to right), because the patient
        will always be reading into a scotoma. Nine o'clock can also be
        difficult because the reader will have difficulty returning to the
        beginning of the next line. Both 12 and 6 o'clock work fairly well
        for reading, with 12 o'clock being slightly better due to the ability
        to see the lines below the one being read.

7. c. The uncorrected myopia simply adds to the power of the microscope resulting in a +19-D system. The viewing distance (focal length) of this system is very close to 2 inches, or about 5.2 cm (the same value, but not the same units as one of the incorrect choices) (1/19 = 0.052; 5.2 cm/2.54 cm/inch = 2 inches).

8. c. Use of the F/4 relationship is based on a 25-cm reference distance and would provide an erroneous value of ×2.5. Dr. Louise Sloan proposed a relationship of F/2.5 that is based upon a 40-cm reference distance that would yield the correct value of ×4. This can be further demonstrated with the use of the general formula: Magnification (M) = reference distance (in meters) × F (lens power in diopters). Here, M = (0.4) (10) = ×4.

9. c. A ×4 Keplerian telescope with a 20-D objective lens would have a +80-D eyepiece lens (M = −F eyepiece/F objective). Focusing on an object that is 25 cm away requires +4 D (1/0.25 M) of vergence to be "borrowed" from the objective lens, creating a telemicroscope. The power of a telemicroscope is the product of the telescope magnification times the power of the lens cap. The power of the adjusted telescope would be (+80 D/+16 D) ×5. Multiplying the power of the adjusted telescope by the 4 D of vergence that was "borrowed" to focus at 25 cm results in a (×5) × 4, or +20-D system. An incorrect answer of +16 D would be selected if the student simply multiplies the base power of the telescope by the vergence of the virtual cap.

10. b. The total height of a 20/20 letter is 8.75 mm. This should be committed to memory. A 20' letter is approximately the same size as a 6-M letter. If this patient moves from 25 cm to 40 cm, the best corrected letter size would increase from 16 M to 25 M. A 25-M letter is about 4 times the size of a 6-M letter. The correct, closest answer is 37.12 mm.

11. c. Application of the inverse-square law reveals that halving the distance would increase the illumination by 4 times. In contrast, doubling the distance would reduce the illumination to 25% of the initial value.

12. c. Telescopes will "amplify" vergence entering the objective approximately by the square of the magnification. Multiplying the +0.5-D lens power by (3^2) 9 results in an approximate value of 4.5 D.

13. c. There are a number of ways of calculating JND. Perhaps the easiest is to take the minimum angle of resolution (MAR) and divide by 10. This would give the value of (MAR = 120/20 = 6) divided by 10 or a JND of ±0.6 D. This value has to be rounded up to the correct answer of ±0.75 D.

14. a. This question is really about aberrations and low vision lenses. Spherical biconvex lenses are inexpensive designs that can exhibit aberrations in higher powers that can affect perceived image quality. Aspheric and aplanatic (air-spaced) doublet lens designs are useful in limiting spherical aberrations and distortion. Achromatic doublets add the benefit of controlling chromatic aberration.

15. c. Contrast sensitivity is the best answer because facial recognition involves primarily central VA and contrast sensitivity. With good acuity, it is reasonable to assume that the difficulty is associated with contrast. Color vision is not necessary for facial recognition (think of black-and-white photographs). Electroretinography (ERG) can isolate problems within the retina; however, given the history of macular degeneration, the ERG is unlikely to be beneficial. A 30-2 threshold Humphrey visual field test will be very difficult for this patient to take and is unlikely to yield useful information. If, however, in the clinical care of this patient the contrast sensitivity was normal, a visual field may be warranted.

16. b. The daily activities of patients with unilateral VA loss will likely not be severely affected. Patients with longstanding bilateral visual field loss will still be able to read and watch television. *Recent* bilateral visual acuity loss is much more likely to be associated with depression than *longstanding* bilateral visual acuity loss, in which a patient has had the opportunity to acknowledge or accept the impairment.

17. d. The size of the telescope exit pupil is determined by dividing the objective lens diameter by the magnification of the telescope. The brightness of an extended object is reduced if the exit pupil of the telescope is smaller than the patient's pupil. Further, the smallest exit pupil, 2 mm in the case of the 4×8 telescope, would constrain image brightness the most.

18. a. Students should be familiar with the relationship: $F_{eq} = F_1 + F_2 - dF_1F_2$, where d is the separation between two lenses, in this case the reading glasses and the hand-held magnifier. When the two lenses are separated by the focal length of the hand-held magnifier (1/8 D) 12.5 cm, dF_1F_2 equals the power of the add and F_{eq} equals the power of the hand-held magnifier.

19. b. The field of view of a lens is directly proportional to the lens diameter and inversely proportional to both the power of the lens and the distance between the lens and the eye. Therefore, increasing the distance between the hand-held magnifier and the eye will reduce field of view.

20. b. By convention, telescopes are labeled as magnification × objective lens diameter. An 8 × 50 telescope has ×8 magnification and a 50-mm objective lens diameter. Further, dividing the entrance pupil diameter (typically the objective lens in a Galilean telescope) by the exit pupil diameter yields the telescope magnification. The telescope described here is (15 mm/5 mm) ×3 and the correct designation is 3 × 15.

21. a. A relatively weak bifocal add can be used with a CCTV, permitting some flexibility in working distance. Consider a +10-D equivalent power with ×4 CCTV magnification and a +2.50 add. A "blur" of 0.25 D would be created by the patient viewing the CCTV about 4 cm closer than 40 cm. However, the same 0.25-D "blur" would be created by a 2.5-mm change in distance for the other three devices.

22. d. Increasing the television size or decreasing viewing distance is the preferable modification. The Fresnel TV magnifiers have optical limitations but are successfully used by many patients. Telescopic devices have limited fields that may prevent visualization of the entire television screen and thus limit the benefits of angular magnification.

23. d. The commonly accepted analogy is that bioptic telescopes are used like rear view mirrors: drivers use them for brief spotting and identification tasks. Most driving tasks can be performed while viewing through the spectacle carrier lens. Actually viewing through the telescope should only occur for a fraction of the time while driving, with 5% being the most logical choice.

24. d. This is a simple two-step question. The first part is to determine the equivalent power required for this patient to read 1-M print. The ratio of test distance/target size is constant and can be used to determine the required equivalent power.

$$\frac{0.4}{4\,M} = \frac{\text{unknown distance}}{1M}$$

Solving for the unknown distance yields 0.1 m, which means the equivalent power is (1/0.1) or 10 D. The second part of this question is to find the telemicroscope that has 10 D of total equivalent power. Because the magnification of a telemicroscope is the product of the angular magnification of the telescope times the power of the reading cap, the correct answer is the ×4 telescope with the +2.5–D cap.

25. a. Denial (sometimes referred to as shock) is the first stage of grieving described by Kübler-Ross. This is followed by anger, depression, bargaining, and eventual acceptance. Although Kübler-Ross was not writing about visual loss, the psychosocial effects in low vision are very similar to the stages of grieving that she described.

26. b. Individuals with oculocutaneous albinism (OCA) typically present with mild to moderate photophobia, reduced visual acuity, and nystagmus. Color vision is normal in OCA patients, unless there is another condition present causing the color vision defect.

27. d. A macular hole produces a small area of central visual deficit with an intact periphery. The other three conditions can cause severe peripheral defects that would impair the ability to drive safely.

28. b. An object that is positioned 5 cm below the lens has (1/–0.05 m) or –20 D of divergence at the plane of the stand magnifier. Using the vergence relationship:

$$L + F = L'$$
$$-10 + 15 = L' = -5 \text{ D}$$

The maximum add power that can be used to view the image would be equal in magnitude, but necessarily opposite in power, to the divergence exiting the stand magnifier, or +5 D.

29. d. Prism for field enhancement is placed with the base in the direction of the field loss over the eye on the same side as the field loss. The image is shifted in the direction of the apex, thus allowing the patient to make a smaller eye movement to see objects in the affected portion of the visual field.

30. d. Each step size of 0.1 logMAR represents about a 1.26 difference in size. The 0.3 logMAR steps equal a $(1.26 \times 1.26 \times 1.26)$ or 2 times size difference, and 0.6 logMAR equals a 4 times size difference, for the correct answer of 20/200.

CHAPTER 30

Sensory Anomalies of Binocular Vision/ Strabismus

John R. Griffin

1. On monocular fixation testing, your amblyopic patient has a negative angle kappa (corneal light reflex displaced temporally from the center of the pupil) in the right eye, but the reflex is central in the pupil of the left eye. The most likely cause of this is:
   a. alternating esotropia
   b. alternating exotropia
   c. unilateral esotropia of the right eye
   d. unilateral exotropia of the right eye

2. A patient with an amblyopic eye with spatial distortion and uncertainty along with errors in direction is most likely to have:
   a. unilateral strabismus with eccentric fixation
   b. unilateral strabismus with central fixation
   c. alternating strabismus with alternating suppression
   d. anisometropia with the ametropia being greater in the amblyopic eye

3. A patient with anisometropic amblyopia of the left eye would likely have _____ when monocularly fixating with that eye.
   a. spatial distortion and a negative angle kappa
   b. eccentric fixation with spatial distortion
   c. central fixation with spatial distortion
   d. central fixation without spatial distortion

4. Testing with visually evoked cortical potential is helpful in cases of reduced visual acuity with suspected amblyopia to determine if the cause is due to an:
   a. unsteady fixation
   b. anomalous correspondence
   c. organic lesion
   d. eccentric fixation

5. Interferometry is useful to prognosticate potential visual acuity of an amblyopic patient and it is:
   a. determined by refractive error
   b. affected by minor opacities of the ocular media
   c. determined by grating orientation reporting
   d. done by determining movement of vertical gratings

6. Interferometry is used for prognostic reasons to predict visual acuity outcomes for _____ following vision therapy.
   a. reduction of eccentric fixation
   b. elimination of anomalous correspondence
   c. evaluation of optokinetic nystagmus visual acuity
   d. improvement of Snellen visual acuity

7. The condition most likely to cause amblyopia would be:
   a. hyperopic anisometropia with alternating exotropia
   b. myopic anisometropia with unilateral exotropia
   c. hyperopic anisometropia with alternating esotropia
   d. hyperopic anisometropia with unilateral esotropia

8. For your amblyopic patient, you provide ophthalmoscopic evaluation and testing of visual fields and color vision, all of which are important for detecting:
   a. unsteady fixation
   b. eccentric fixation
   c. ocular disease
   d. suppression

9. Your patient has amblyopia of the left eye with an angle kappa of −1 mm. The patient has 20/20 (6/6) acuity in the right eye with an angle kappa of +1 mm. The deviation of the left eye in this case is:
   a. nasal eccentric fixation
   b. temporal eccentric fixation
   c. esotropia
   d. exotropia

10. Case history is important prognostically for patients with amblyopia. Generally, the most important consideration is:
    a. whether the deviation was esotropic or exotropic
    b. whether the refractive error was myopic or hyperopic
    c. the time or onset and time and duration of vision therapy
    d. whether the strabismus was constant or intermittent

11. Tests such as Hess-Lancaster, von Graefe with vertical prism displacement, and Maddox rod can be used to determine the angle of:
    a. anomaly
    b. eccentric fixation
    c. subjective directionalization
    d. objective angle of the deviation of the visual axes

12. A red Maddox rod is placed before the patient's right eye. Even if suppression is deep, this "unnatural" test would most likely overcome the suppression. A vertical red streak is reported to be seen to the left of the penlight target. This indicates the patient has an:
    a. exotropia
    b. esotropia
    c. esodeviation of the visual axes
    d. exodeviation of the visual axes

13. In strabismus, suppression is a defense against:
    a. pathologic diplopia
    b. physiologic diplopia
    c. confusion
    d. confusion and diplopia

14. The cause of pathologic diplopia in a case of strabismus is due to:
    a. noncorresponding points of the peripheral retina being stimulated by one target
    b. corresponding points of the peripheral retina being stimulated by one target
    c. the fovea of each eye being stimulated by two targets
    d. the fovea of one eye being stimulated by two targets

15. In strabismus the suppression usually occurs first at the:
    a. target point (point "zero") of the deviating eye
    b. target point (point "zero") of the fixating eye
    c. fovea of the deviating eye
    d. fovea of the fixating eye

16. A suppression is more intense ("deeper") if it is shown on testing with:
     a. vectograms
     b. septa such as a bar reader
     c. septa with optical systems, as a Brewster stereoscope
     d. colored filters as on the Worth four-dot test

17. Suppression in cases of anisometropia is usually _____ because of only the _____ area being involved.
     a. large, foveal
     b. small, foveal
     c. large, point zero
     d. small, point zero

18. Anomalous correspondence, clinically often referred to as anomalous *retinal* correspondence (ARC), occurs when there is an angle of anomaly. This angle would be _____ prism diopters in a strabismic patient with 20 prism diopters of esotropia but reports seeing as though orthophoric on testing with a major amblyoscope.
     a. 0
     b. 10
     c. 20
     d. 30

19. On the cover test with prisms, you measure 15 prism diopters of esotropia and an orthophoric response with Maddox rod testing. This indicates _____ correspondence.
     a. normal
     b. harmonious anomalous
     c. typical unharmonious anomalous
     d. paradoxical anomalous

20. You have an esotropic patient with an objective angle of 20 prism diopters but the subjective angle is only 10 prism diopters of esodeviation. This indicates _____ correspondence.
     a. normal
     b. harmonious anomalous
     c. typical unharmonious anomalous
     d. paradoxical anomalous

21. You have another patient with an esotropia of 20 prism diopters (objective angle) but the subjective angle is a 10-prism-diopter exodeviation. This indicates _____ correspondence.
     a. normal
     b. harmonious anomalous
     c. typical unharmonious anomalous
     d. paradoxical type one anomalous

22. You have a patient with 20 prism diopters of esotropia of the right eye. There is harmonious anomalous correspondence. The Hering-Bielschowsky afterimage is given. The fovea of the fixating left eye is flashed with a horizontal streak and the fovea of the deviating right eye is flashed with a vertical streak (each eye under monocular seeing conditions). With both eyes open, the patient reports seeing afterimages with the vertical streak being:
    a. 20 prism diopters to the left of the horizontal streak
    b. 20 prism diopters to the right of the horizontal streak
    c. 10 prism diopters to the right of the horizontal streak
    d. in the center of the horizontal streak (perfect cross)

23. You have a strabismic patient who is unable to achieve superimposition of haploscopically presented targets in a major amblyoscope (e.g., synoptophore). The targets may appear to jump past each other as they are moved in the instrument to approach each other. This binocular anomaly is known as:
    a. retinal rivalry
    b. intermittent suppression
    c. horror fusionis
    d. harmonious anomalous correspondence

24. There are two main theories for the etiology of anomalous correspondence. One of them is that of Burian. This is thought to be:
    a. sensory adaptation to strabismus
    b. a motor phenomenon involving innervation to the extraocular muscles
    c. covariation in which the angle of anomaly decreases with the decreasing angle of strabismus
    d. the all-or-none concept in which the correspondence is sometimes normal and sometimes abnormal

25. Onset of anomalous correspondence is usually before the age of _____ years and rarely after the age of _____ years.
    a. 6, 15
    b. 9, 18
    c. 12, 21
    d. 15, 24

26. The most prevalent type of anomalous correspondence is:
    a. unharmonious
    b. harmonious
    c. paradoxical type one
    d. paradoxical type two

27. Some clinical tests such as _____ are more likely to reveal harmonious rather than unharmonious anomalous correspondence.
    a. major amblyoscope measurements and afterimages
    b. Bagolini striated lenses and free-space diplopia testing
    c. Maddox rod with cover test and Bagolini striated lenses
    d. major amblyoscope measurements and free-space diplopia testing

28. When an individual fixates on a distant object while holding a pencil at a nearpoint in the midline, the pencil will appear to be double unless there is _____ suppression and the diplopia will be _____.
    a. physiologic, heteronymous
    b. physiologic, homonymous
    c. pathologic, heteronymous
    d. pathologic, homonymous

29. Central suppression in strabismic individuals is needed to prevent _____, and peripheral suppression is needed to prevent _____.
    a. diplopia, confusion
    b. anomalous correspondence of the harmonious type
    c. diplopia, horror fusionis
    d. confusion, diplopia

30. When testing for superimposition ("first-degree fusion") using a major amblyoscope (e.g., synoptophore) and superimposition cannot be attained, there is either _____ or _____ present.
    a. pathologic suppression, horror fusionis
    b. horror fusionis, lack of correspondence
    c. physiologic suppression, lack of correspondence
    d. physiologic suppression, horror fusionis

31. Worth classified sensory fusion into four levels. The level at which most clinical testing is performed to evaluate motor fusion is:
    a. simultaneous perception
    b. superimposition
    c. flat fusion
    d. stereopsis

32. Tests of stereopsis may include check marks as suppression clues. A way that you can use such stereopsis targets to evaluate the effects of fusional vergence on stereopsis while monitoring for suppression is by having the patient report that:
    a. one checkmark disappears
    b. both checkmarks disappear
    c. the fused target is seen in depth before it is seen as diplopic
    d. perception of depth diminishes, although the checkmarks may remain visible

33. As regards stereoacuity, your patient would rank as _____ if testing results indicate 100 seconds of arc using a test such as the "reindeer."
    a. weak
    b. adequate
    c. strong
    d. very strong

34. Emile Javal, "father of orthoptics," treated strabismus in the late 1800s, and one of his first principles was to _____, and then _____, followed by _____.
    a. treat amblyopia, correct significant refractive error, give antisuppression training
    b. give antisuppression training, correct significant refractive error, treat amblyopia
    c. correct significant refractive error, treat amblyopia, give antisuppression training
    d. correct significant refractive error, give antisuppression training, treat amblyopia

35. In an esotropic patient with harmonious anomalous correspondence, the sequence of therapy to be advised is treatment for:
    a. amblyopia, suppression, anomalous correspondence
    b. anomalous correspondence, amblyopia, suppression
    c. suppression, amblyopia, suppression
    d. amblyopia, anomalous correspondence, suppression

36. Your patient is 18 years old and has intermittent exotropia with harmonious anomalous correspondence when the deviation is manifest. Occlusion of an eye is a technique that can be used to treat the anomalous correspondence because there is no anomalous correspondence in play under monocular viewing conditions. A reason why occlusion would not be advised in this case is because:
    a. the intermittent exotropia could become a constant exotropia with prolonged occlusion
    b. occlusion is an antisuppression technique
    c. the anomalous correspondence becomes more embedded when the eyes are in the heterotropic position
    d. horror fusionis would result

37. Your 9-year-old patient has intermittent exotropia of 12 prism diopters with harmonious exotropia when the deviation is manifest. As regards prism correction, the initial choice for prescription would be:
    a. 12 prism diopters base-in
    b. 12 prism diopters base-out
    c. 24 prism diopters base-in
    d. no prism prescription

38. Your 21-year-old patient recently had extraocular muscle surgery for 25 prism diopters of constant unilateral esotropia with harmonious anomalous correspondence. Postsurgically, the patient has 6 prism diopters of constant unilateral esotropia with unharmonious anomalous correspondence. The recommendation of choice in this case is to:
    a. prescribe 6 prism diopters base-in
    b. prescribe 6 prism diopters base-out
    c. give antisuppression training in the hope of attaining sensory fusion
    d. give no optical or training prescription

39. Your 6-year-old patient with an exodeviation has a very large refractive anisometropia due to each eye having different corneal curvatures. This results in suppression of an eye and, consequently, intermittent exotropia of the suppressing eye. The best prescription that would likely be the best choice to consider in this case is:
    a. iseikonic-size lenses
    b. contact lenses
    c. spectacles with full correction of the ametropia of each eye
    d. keratorefractive surgery

40. Home training instruments such as television trainers, Pola-mirror, and reading bars are designed especially for treating:
    a. amblyopia
    b. anomalous correspondence
    c. suppression
    d. poor stereopsis

41. In pediatric screening for stereopsis, most children can detect stereopsis when viewing the Randot preschool stereoacuity test as early as the age of _____.
    a. 1 year
    b. 2 years
    c. 4 years
    d. 6 years

42. In vision training of a heterophoric patient, the sensory anomaly of suppression can most likely be monitored during binocular lens rock with plus and minus lenses using:
    a. bar readers
    b. Hart charts
    c. Ann Arbor (Michigan tracking)
    d. Marsden ball

43. Your 12-year-old patient has a small-angle esotropia of the right eye of 3 prism diopters. You will likely find upon testing that the patient has _____.
   a. central suppression
   b. amblyopia
   c. gross peripheral fusion
   d. central suppression, amblyopia, gross peripheral fusion

44. The well-known methods of Bangerter and Cuppers are for _____ in cases of _____.
   a. pleoptics, amblyopia with eccentric fixation
   b. pleoptics, amblyopia with central fixation
   c. orthoptics, anomalous correspondence
   d. orthoptics, suppression

45. The oldest, most used, and effective treatment of amblyopia is:
   a. direct occlusion
   b. indirect occlusion
   c. direct occlusion and monocular fixation training
   d. indirect occlusion and monocular fixation training

Answers

1. c. Unilateral esotropia of the right eye of long duration can result in amblyopia with nasal eccentric fixation, with a negative angle kappa on monocular testing of the amblyopic eye.

2. a. The weight of authority holds that eccentric fixation causes the spatial visual problems in strabismic amblyopia. Eccentric fixation is less prevalent in anisometropic amblyopia.

3. d. There is usually central fixation in an amblyopic eye caused by anisometropia. Fixation may be unsteady, but spatial distortion is relatively little compared with a strabismic, amblyopic eye with eccentric fixation.

4. c. Reduced VECP amplitude may indicate optic atrophy, and latency differences may indicate optic nerve demyelination as in multiple sclerosis.

5. c. Resolution acuity of spatial frequency of line gratings in an interferometer corresponding to Snellen visual acuity is usually not greatly affected by opacities or refractive errors. The patient is asked to tell which way the lines are slanted.

6. d. Interferometry helps in predicting posttherapy visual acuity. Optokinetic nystagmus, although usually better than Snellen acuity, is not as reliable in predicting posttherapy visual acuity.

7. d. Both anisometropia, especially hyperopic, and unilateral esotropia are amblyogenic. Unilateral exotropia is usually less amblyogenic because it tends to be more intermittent than unilateral esotropia; the person intermittently would have the possible opportunity to fuse images binocularly, thus stimulating the amblyopic eye to be used during bifixation.

8. c. It is always important to rule out ocular disease that reduces visual acuity for making a differential diagnosis from functional amblyopia.

9. a. Remember that reliable angle kappa testing, as opposed to binocular Hirschberg testing, is performed monocularly. The left eye with angle kappa of −1 mm means that the eye turn is nasalward with the target image falling on an eccentric point nasal to the fovea.

10. c. The time of onset and the length of time between onset and beginning of vision therapy are crucial. For example, even if the onset is at age 1 year, the prognosis for functional cure can be good if therapy is begun immediately. If more than 7 years pass before therapy, the prognosis would be poor. Intermittency of strabismus is an important consideration also, but many patients with amblyopia have anisometropia, and history of strabismus alone is insufficient as regards prognosis.

11. c. The above tests depend on subjective responses of the patient. The objective angle is measured by the cover test, Hirschberg, and other such procedures from the examiner's view. Eccentric fixation is measured monocularly. The angle of anomaly depends on the relationship between the subjective and objective angles.

12. d. The right eye is in the exo posture in relation to the light, which causes "crossed diplopia." The doctor cannot differentiate between a heterophoria and heterotropia using only this subjective test.

13. d. Diplopia in strabismus is considered to be "pathologic" and confusion results when the fovea of each eye is directed toward different targets. Suppression helps the individual avoid these disturbing annoyances.

14. a. Unless there is suppression or compensating angle of anomaly, stimulation of noncorresponding points results in diplopia.

15. c. Most strabismic patients do not complain of confusion as much as diplopia, indicating the fovea is more quickly and intensely suppressed than a point zero in the peripheral retina.

16. d. Targets with colored filters such as the red and green on the Worth four-dot test are very unnatural and less likely to detect a shallow suppression than would a more natural test such as a vectogram.

17. b. Assuming the patient's eyes are mostly in the ortho position because of adequate peripheral fusion, point zero (target point) of each eye is at the fovea of each eye, making a central suppression small.

18. c. The angle of anomaly is measured by subtracting the subjective angle of directionalization from the objective angle of strabismus. In this case it is 20 − 0 = 20.

19. b. Harmonious correspondence is indicated when the objective angle of strabismus and the angle of anomaly are of the same magnitude. Orthophoric position is simulated; this is not true fusion because the fovea of the fixating eye is corresponding with a peripheral point (or small area) of the retina of the deviating eye.

20. c. The angle of strabismus is larger than the subjective angle and the angle of anomaly. This is the typical type of unharmonious correspondence.

21. d. This atypical type of disharmony where the objective and subjective angles are in opposite direction is the paradoxical type one anomalous correspondence.

22. a. The fovea of the esotropic left eye is temporal to the anomalous point that corresponds with the fovea of the left eye. The vertical afterimage would be seen as though projected to the left of the horizontal afterimage. Note that the anomalous point is at the same location as point zero in the right eye, because of the harmonious type of anomalous correspondence in this case.

23. c. This anomaly is explained by Flom's horopter theory in which there is a notch centrally in the identical visual direction horopter, creating relative distribution of corresponding points without uniformity.

24. a. Burian presented the sensory concept of depth of anomalous correspondence, which is analogous to depth of suppression ranging from shallow to deep. Strabismus would cause the anomalous correspondence as an adaptation to the deviation of the visual axes.

25. a. Most strabismic children with anomalous correspondence had onset of it in the early developmental years. It is rare to have anomalous correspondence beginning in teenagers or adults.

26. b. Harmonious anomalous correspondence allows for some rudimentary degree of binocular vision and elimination of diplopia. When normal correspondence is not attainable because of the strabismic deviation, the next best choice is harmonious anomalous correspondence.

27. b. The more unnatural tests, such as the Maddox rod or major amblyoscopes, tend to reveal unharmonious anomalous correspondence more so than relatively more natural tests such as free-space diplopia testing and Bagolini striated lenses.

28.   a.   If the individual can release the physiologic suppression, the pencil will be perceived with heteronymous ("crossed") diplopia.

29.   d.   The foveal image of the deviating eye must be suppressed to avoid confusion, and the peripheral image must be suppressed to avoid diplopia.

30.   b.   Unless there is a lack of any correspondence, images can be directionally perceived and suppression can almost always be broken in such an unnatural environment as in a major amblyoscope that has color and brightness contrast and intermittent illuminated stimuli. Images can be directionally perceived in horror fusionis as close as being side by side but not superimposed.

31.   c.   Flat fusion ("second-degree fusion") is the integration of two similar ocular images into a single percept. It is used, for example, generally to measure fusional divergence and convergence ranges. The targets often incorporate unfusible checkmarks as suppression clues.

32.   d.   The quality of stereopsis is affected by blur, which can occur with motor fusional demands as well as suppression occurring under the stress.

33.   a.   Adequate stereoacuity would be in the range of 31 to 60 seconds of arc using a test with contours and of 51 to 100 using noncontoured targets such as random dots. In this case, 100 seconds of arc on a contoured target is not adequate and is considered "weak."

34.   c.   Good visual acuity in each eye is important for vision therapy to be successful. Correction of any significant refractive error is the first step. Likewise, amblyopia should be abated to afford good acuity in each eye. After that, binocular therapy with antisuppression training can then be considered.

35.   d.   Amblyopia is one of the first considerations as visual acuity is most important. Because anomalous correspondence is antidiplopic for the patient, antisuppression training could possibly result with the patient having intractable diplopia, unless normal correspondence is achieved.

36.   a.   Occlusion disrupts fusion, causing the latent exodeviation to become manifest more frequently, and because of covariation, the anomalous correspondence becomes manifest more frequently. If the strabismus becomes constant, the anomalous correspondence would be present 100% of the time.

37. d. Because of covariation, there may be normal correspondence when the patient is fusing in the ortho position. Fusional convergence training is the best choice in the beginning of therapy. Relieving base-in prism of low power can later be considered, if necessary, after normal correspondence is well established and the patient has bifixation most of the time.

38. d. Assuming there is no cosmetic problem with the small-angle strabismus and there is suppression sufficient to prevent diplopia, it is wise to forego therapy. Breaking suppression in this case could result in the patient having intractable diplopia.

39. b. Spectacle lenses may cause aniseikonia and create difficulties for the patient. Iseikonic-size lenses could be considered in the future if absolutely necessary. Surgery would not be advised initially in this young patient. Contact lenses would minimize aniseikonia, according to Knapp's law. If there is amblyopia, spectacle lenses with full correction of the amblyopia eye would be given, mainly for monocular vision training activities. Contact lenses, however, allow for bifoveal fusion, which can abate amblyopia providing central suppression is addressed.

40. c. Suppression can also be monitored while fusional vergence demands are introduced. The suppression clue with the television trainer is a portion of the video screen being invisible; a suppressing eye is invisible with the Pola-mirror; some words are not seen by the suppressing eye with reading bars.

41. b. This is likely when using Book No. 3 with stereoacuity thresholds of 400 to 800 seconds of arc.

42. a. Bar readers are good for checking suppression, and even foveal suppression when viewing words of small font. The other options have monocular demands, but they can be binocular with suppression monitoring, as with red and green lettering while wearing red-green filters.

43. d. There are numerous terms for this condition, such as monofixational syndrome, microtropia, fusion disparity, monofixational esophoria, retinal flicker, microtropia unilateralis, and anomalofusionalis. Note that eccentric fixation and harmonious anomalous correspondence are also typically found in these cases.

44. a. The term "pleoptics" generally refers to therapy for amblyopia with eccentric fixation.

45. c. "Indirect occlusion" refers to patching the amblyopic eye as part of a pleoptics regimen. Although it is possible to have favorable treatment results, this form of therapy is seldom used.

Anomalies of Eye Movements

John R. Griffin

1. Eye movements that are fast and voluntary and suppress ocular images during movement are most likely to be:
    a. pursuits
    b. saccade
    c. vergences
    d. vestibule-ocular movements

2. The developmental eye movement test (DEM) is similar to the King-Devick test, except that it:
    a. is a subjective test
    b. measures saccadic eye movements
    c. accounts for rapid automatic naming
    d. is a series of numbers on cards presented to the patient

3. You have a 20-year-old male patient who has a small intermittent esotropia in the primary position, and the deviation increases on left gaze. You suspect paresis of the:
    a. right lateral rectus
    b. left lateral rectus
    c. left medial rectus
    d. right medial rectus

4. A patient with a paretic left lateral rectus muscle probably would have an abnormal head position that is a _____ to the _____.
    a. tilt, left
    b. tilt, right
    c. turn, left
    d. turn, right

5. You have a 32-year-old female patient who recently was in an automobile accident. Upon examination, there is a small hypertropia of the right eye in the primary position of gaze. On left gaze the hypertropia becomes larger, and it is greatest on right head tilt. The affected extraocular muscle would likely be the:
    a. left superior oblique
    b. right superior rectus
    c. left superior rectus
    d. right superior oblique

6. A case of a patient with a paretic right superior oblique muscle presents with an increased hypertropia of the right eye on left gaze. There are three other isolated muscles with paresis that could also cause either a hypertropia or a hyperphoria of the right eye in the primary position of gaze. These are the:
    a. right inferior rectus, left inferior rectus, left superior rectus
    b. left inferior oblique, right inferior rectus, left superior rectus
    c. right inferior oblique, right inferior rectus, right superior rectus
    d. right inferior rectus, left inferior rectus, right superior rectus

7. Your patient is a 9-year-old boy. He has a constant, unilateral esotropia of the right eye of 12 prism diopters. You perform the unilateral cover test (cover-uncover test) and expect to see that the _____:
    a. right eye moves inward when it is covered
    b. left eye moves outward when the right eye is covered
    c. right eye moves outward when it is covered
    d. left eye moves inward when it is covered

8. You want to see if the magnitude of the esodeviation of a patient is the same whether the right eye fixates or the left eye fixates. You can measure this precisely with the alternate cover test and prisms. To do this, the set-up would be to have the left eye, for example, fixating the target and a prism placed:
    a. base-out before the right eye and behind the occluder
    b. base-in before the right eye and behind the occluder
    c. base-out before the unoccluded left eye with the right eye unoccluded
    d. base-in before the unoccluded left eye with the right eye unoccluded

9. You have a patient who is 50 years old and you notice an abnormal head posture as he enters the examination room. His head is turned to the left, tilted with chin down, and tilting toward his left shoulder. You suspect that you will find a paretic _____ extraocular muscle.
    a. left superior oblique
    b. left superior rectus
    c. right superior rectus
    d. right superior oblique

10. Your patient has a history of infantile esotropia with a constant, unilateral esotropia of 6 prism diopters. On the unilateral cover test you notice that the covered eye drifts upward, but it slowly moves back down after the cover is removed. The same occurrence takes place when the other eye is occluded. You suspect:
    a. Brown syndrome
    b. A or V syndromes
    c. latent hyperphoria
    d. dissociated vertical deviation

11. You have a 4-year-old patient who has had the following condition since birth. There is limited abduction of each eye but only slightly limited adduction of the eyes. There is narrowing of the palpebral fissure of each eye on adduction. The suspected diagnosis is:
    a. paretic medial rectus muscles
    b. Duane syndrome, type 1
    c. Duane syndrome, type 2
    d. Duane syndrome, type 3

12. You have a 7-year-old patient who has hypotropia of the right eye when looking up and to her left side. On duction (monocular) testing, the right eye has limited elevation when it is adducted. The probable diagnosis is:
    a. Duane syndrome, type 1
    b. paretic right inferior oblique
    c. primary overaction of the right inferior oblique
    d. Brown syndrome

13. Fixation disparity is a slight manifest misalignment of the visual axes, measured in _____ and there is _____ and _____ binocular vision.
    a. seconds of arc, sensory fusion, diplopic
    b. minutes of arc, central suppression, single
    c. seconds of arc, sensory fusion, single
    d. minutes of arc, sensory fusion, single

14. A test for fixation disparity, such as the Saladin near point balance card is used to measure directly the angle of fixation disparity in _____ and the associated phoria (neutralizing power) that is measured in _____.
    a. degrees, spherical diopters
    b. minutes, spherical diopters
    c. seconds, prism diopters
    d. minutes, prism diopters

15. You have a symptomatic patient who has an esofixation disparity of 4 minutes of arc with an associated phoria of 8 prism diopters base-out and a motor fusion range of 3 base-in to 11 base-out breakpoints. From this information alone, the vergence anomaly that this patient has is probably:
    a. divergence insufficiency
    b. divergence excess
    c. convergence insufficiency
    d. convergence excess

16. Tentatively, the prescription for vision therapy for a patient with convergence excess would be:
    a. plus-addition adds for reading
    b. base-out fusion training and plus-addition adds for reading
    c. base-in fusion training
    d. base-in fusion training and plus-addition adds for reading

17. Testing to determine if an underacting extraocular muscle is due to a paresis or to a restricting, anatomical cause can be done by using _____ test.
    a. the forced duction
    b. the Hirschberg
    c. the alternate cover
    d. a red-green dissociation

18. You have an uncooperative young patient who is restless and resists cover testing and wearing of red-green filters. The Hirschberg test, however, is accepted by the patient. The patient has fusion in all diagnostic positions of gaze. Noncomitancy could be most likely be determined by estimating the magnitudes of the:
    a. primary deviations with prisms
    b. secondary deviations without prisms
    c. deviation in various positions of gaze by disrupting fusion by having the child look through a base-down prism before an eye
    d. deviation by direct observation as the child is asked to look at various objects of interest in the room

19. Vergence facility is measured by step vergence responses to base-in and base-out prismatic demands. Most commonly used as performance criteria with suppression monitoring are powers for distant viewing of _____ and _____ for near viewing for a time period of _____.
    a. 4 base-in to 8 base-out, 8 base-in and 8 base-out, 1 minute
    b. 4 base-in to 8 base-out, 8 base-in to 8 base-out, 1.5 minutes
    c. 4 base-in to 4 base-out, 4 base-in to 8 base-out, 2 minutes
    d. 8 base-in to 12 base-out, 12 base-in to 12 base-out, 2.5 minutes

20. A patient with adequate vergence facility should normally have at least _____ cycles per minute with clear, single vision with suppression being monitored.
   a. 1
   b. 5
   c. 10
   d. 15

21. You see a patient with nystagmus characterized by vision under binocular conditions being better than monocular. The patient has infantile esotropia. You suspect:
   a. ocillopsia
   b. manifest nystagmus
   c. latent nystagmus
   d. sensory nystagmus

22. Possible optical therapy for manifest motor nystagmus is to prescribe _____ for near viewing or _____ for both near and far viewing.
   a. minus addition lenses, base-in prisms
   b. plus addition lenses, base-out prisms
   c. minus addition lenses, base-out prisms
   d. plus addition lenses, base-in prisms

23. The alternate cover test is especially valuable in determining:
   a. the frequency of strabismus
   b. which eye is dominant and preferred for fixation
   c. cosmesis of strabismus
   d. magnitude of the deviation of the visual axes

24. Very small manifest strabismic angles can be detected with the Brückner test. The light reflex in a case of unilateral esotropia of the left eye will appear to be _____ in the strabismic eye.
   a. displaced temporally (templeward)
   b. displaced nasally (nasalward)
   c. dimmer
   d. brighter

25. Dextrosupraversion, levosupraversion, dextroinfraversion, and levoinfraversion are _____ diagnostic positions of gaze of which there are _____ other diagnostic positions of gaze.
   a. tertiary, three
   b. tertiary, five
   c. secondary, three
   d. secondary, five

Answers

1. b. Saccades are relatively fast with abrupt shifts in fixation and mainly voluntary and suppress the ocular images during movement.

2. c. The DEM has vertical columns of numbers as well as horizontal rows of numbers. Rapid automatic naming is more likely to be evaluated with the vertical array of regularly spaced targets than with horizontal rows of numbers that are irregularly spaced. If the patient performs poorly on the horizontal display, differential diagnosis can be made as to the fault being either to poor saccadic eye movements (as in reading) or to slow random automatic naming, or to both causes.

3. b. A paretic left lateral rectus would cause this noncomitancy. The esodeviation would increase because abduction is limited in the left eye due to its paretic lateral rectus.

4. c. A tilt means the heads tilt toward a shoulder. This patient would have a head turn to his left side. The rule is that the face turn is in the direction of the diagnostic action field of the paretic muscle.

5. d. The three-step method for identifying a paretic cyclovertical muscle can be applied here. One of the actions of the superior oblique is infraduction. Paresis of the right superior oblique muscle could explain the hypertropia of the right eye in the primary position of gaze.

6. b. The inferior oblique elevates. A paretic left inferior oblique would cause a left hypodeviation, making a relative hyperdeviation of the right eye. The inferior rectus depresses. A paretic right inferior rectus would result in a hyperdeviation in that eye. The superior rectus elevates. A paretic left superior rectus would result in an hypodeviation of that eye, thus, a relative hyperdeviation of the right eye.

7. d. When the fixating left eye is covered, the right eye moves outward to take up fixation. The conjugate movement of the eyes results in the left eye moving inward behind the cover.

8. a. Prism is used to neutralize the esodeviation. The prism is placed between the right eye and the occluder; otherwise, prism adaptation could take place if both eyes are left unoccluded. To measure the deviation with the right eye fixating, the prism is placed between the left eye and the occluder.

9. d. A general rule as regards abnormal head posture is that the
        patient's face points in the same direction as the diagnostic action
        field of the affected muscle. In this case of the right superior
        oblique, its diagnostic action field is down and to the left. This is
        where the main action is depression and horizontal and torsional
        effects are minimized. According to the rule, his face would be
        pointed down and to his left side. The head tilt would be to his left
        because the underacting right superior oblique insufficiently intorts
        the eye. To be sure of your clinical hypothesis, you apply the head
        tilt (Bielschowsky) test and find an increased hyperdeviation on
        right head tilt and no noticeable effect on left head tilt.

10. d. Although the etiology is not known for sure, dissociated vertical
        deviation (DVD) is not uncommon. Occasionally you can see
        excycloduction and latent nystagmus when the eye elevates.
        Although surgery may be beneficial in some cases of DVD, you
        would probably not recommend that therapy, unless there were
        symptomatic or cosmetic concerns.

11. b. This is the classic and most prevalent of the three basic types
        of Duane syndrome. The etiology may be due to paradoxical
        innervation in which there is co-contraction of the medial and
        lateral muscles.

12. d. This has also been called a superior tendon sheath syndrome,
        because a mechanical restriction of elevation on adduction
        involving the sheath of superior oblique muscle would cause the
        syndrome, but there are other possible etiologies that give a similar
        effect. For example, a paretic inferior oblique of the right eye
        would cause hypotropia on up and left gaze, although there would
        be no restriction on a forced duction test.

13. d. There is usually central sensory fusion without suppression,
        although the visual axes are slightly (minutes of arc) misaligned
        under binocular viewing conditions.

14. d. Direct measurement of the angle of fixation disparity (angle F) can
        be measured using vernier fiducials by means of crossed polarizing
        filters. The associated phoria of fixation disparity is measured in
        prism diopters while the patient is fusing a target without central
        suppression.

15. d. Assuming testing is performed at near, the patient definitely has an eso problem at near judging by the esofixation disparity, eso-associated phoria, and a steep forced vergence curve considering the limited motor fusion range. Because there were no symptoms reported with distant viewing, there seems to be no farpoint problem; if so, this rules out the farpoint classifications of divergence insufficiency and divergence excess. Convergence excess is the most likely diagnosis until further clinical testing is completed.

16. d. Vision therapy includes several modes of therapy, including optical methods. Plus lenses for reading relieve the eso condition and base-in fusion training help cope with the esophoria. Perhaps vision training can help flatten the slope of the forced vergence curve by expanding the motor fusion range.

17. a. The forced duction test would show an anatomical restriction if rotation of the eye is limited in a diagnostic action field. An innervational etiology, however, would probably show no restriction on forced duction testing.

18. c. The Hirschberg test does not apply to latent deviations, only to manifest deviations of the visual axes, as in strabismus. This patient fuses in the diagnostic positions of gaze and must be made "artificially strabismic" so that the deviation is manifest during the brief moments of Hirschberg testing. Changes in the magnitude of deviation can then be observed.

19. a. Suppression can be monitored with vectograms containing Snellen letters seen exclusively by each eye. One minute is sufficient time to assess speed of the step vergences presented by using flippers with prisms.

20. b. Adequate vergence facility, at either 6 meters or 40 centimeters viewing distance, with standard prism demands requires at least five cycles (10 presentations) of prism rock.

21. c. Nystagmus increases on occlusion of an eye in latent nystagmus. This type is often associated with infantile esotropia.

22. b. For some patients, the nystagmus may be dampened by the act of fusional convergence. This demand can indirectly be introduced with plus addition lenses for near, or directly with base-out prisms creating demands on fusional convergence.

23.   d.   Magnitude of the deviation can be measured with a prism during
           alternate cover testing. Different magnitudes in different directions
           of gaze indicate noncomitancy, which could suggest serious health
           issues.

24.   d.   The red reflex of the deviated eye appears brighter than that of the
           fixating eye. There is no displacement of the red reflex, but there is
           a displacement of the corneal reflex, as in the less-sensitive
           Hirschberg test.

25.   b.   The other diagnostic positions are the primary (straight ahead) and
           the secondary (left, right, up, down) directions of gaze.

CHAPTER 32

Anomalies of Accommodation and Accommodative Vergence

John R. Griffin

1. The monocular estimate method (MEM) can be used to measure accommodative lag. A lag of 0.75D would be ranked as _____ and an accommodative excess of 0.75D would be ranked as _____.
    a. good, adequate
    b. adequate, very poor
    c. poor, adequate
    d. very poor, good

2. The amplitude of accommodation is measured _____ and is referred to as _____ accommodation.
    a. monocularly, relative
    b. binocularly, relative
    c. monocularly, absolute
    d. binocularly, absolute

3. There are several testing procedures for measuring accommodative facility. The most commonly used spherical lens powers are +2.00 and −2.00 diopters held in a flipper holder. Adequate binocular accommodative facility testing with suppression monitoring is _____ cycles per minute and monocular testing would yield _____ cycles per minute.
    a. 6 to 7, more
    b. 6 to 7, less
    c. 8 to 10, more
    d. 8 to 10, less

4. There are several ways to determine the accommodative-convergence/
    accommodation (AC/A) ratio. Using the gradient method, the AC/A
    ratio is _____ if the patient has exophoria of 5 prism diopters at near
    (40 cm) and 10 prism diopters at the same distance when measured
    through a +1.00D lens.
    a. 1/1
    b. 5/1
    c. 10/1
    d. 15/1

5. A graphical method can be used to determine an AC/A ratio by
    inspecting the slope of the phoria line. Assuming the interpupillary
    distance (IPD) is 6 cm, the vergence demand line would have a 6/1
    slope. The phoria line is plotted using the far and near heterophoria
    measurements taken through a phoropter. An exodeviation that is equal
    at far and near would have the phoria line that is to the _____ the
    demand line and an exodeviation that is more exo at near would have
    the phoria line with a _____ steep slope than the demand line.
    a. right and parallel to, more
    b. left and parallel to, less
    c. right and not parallel to, more
    d. left and not parallel to, less

6. Your 11-year-old patient has esophoria of 2 prism diopters at 6 meters
    and 12 prism diopters at 40 centimeters. The chief complaint is blurring
    and discomfort when reading and doing near work. The calculated AC/A
    ratio is _____. This type of vergence anomaly is most likely a case
    of _____.
    a. 8/1, divergence insufficiency
    b. 8/1, convergence excess
    c. 10/1, divergence insufficiency
    d. 10/1, convergence excess

7. The optical treatment you would initially consider for young patients with
    convergence excess is _____ additions in the form of _____ lenses.
    a. plus, single vision
    b. minus, bifocal
    c. plus, bifocal
    d. minus, single vision

8. If your patient with convergence excess has a 10/1 AC/A ratio, an
    addition of +1.50D would theoretically reduce an esodeviation at near of
    12 prism diopters to _____ prism diopters.
    a. esophoria of 3
    b. esophoria of 0
    c. exophoria of 3
    d. exophoria of 5

9. The purpose of vision therapy for a patient with convergence excess is to increase fusional divergence skills. A recommended sequence of vision training would likely be as follows:
   a. pencil pushups, aperture-rule trainer, orthopic fusion
   b. orthopic fusion, aperture-rule trainer, pencil pushups
   c. aperture-rule trainer, pencil pushups, orthopic fusion
   d. pencil pushups, orthopic fusion, aperture-rule trainer

10. For patients with convergence excess, pencil pushup training can be recommended to improve _____ convergence, because of the _____ AC/A ratio.
    a. fusional divergence, low
    b. fusional divergence, high
    c. proximal convergence, low
    d. accommodative convergence, high

11. Your patient is able to fuse the largest, farthest red and blue dots at a distance of 7 centimeters from the spectacle plane, which is at the bridge of the nose of this patient. The patient's interpupillary distance (IPD) is 60 millimeters. The absolute convergence response is approximately _____ prism diopters.
    a. 32
    b. 42
    c. 52
    d. 62

12. In cases of convergence insufficiency, the concept of moving the fixation target from far to near applies in vision training since the slope of the AC/A line is _____ than the slope of the demand line. Therefore, the function being trained for improvement is _____ convergence.
    a. less, fusional
    b. more, fusional
    c. less, accommodative
    d. more, accommodative

13. The Vodnoy aperture-rule trainer can be used in cases of convergence insufficiency, with the goal of improving _____ vergence while not viewing targets in an open environment, as in _____ fusion training for these patients.
    a. positive fusional, chiastopic
    b. positive accommodative, chiastopic
    c. negative fusional, orthopic
    d. relative accommodative, orthopic

14. You have a patient who is beginning to master card number 4 on the Vodnoy aperture-rule trainer. The card is viewed from a distance of 40 centimeters. A convenient rule to know the prismatic demand on vergence is to multiply the card number by a factor of 2.5, resulting in 10 prism diopters of vergence demand in this example. This means that the two targets to be fused are separated by _____ centimeters.
   a. 2
   b. 4
   c. 8
   d. 10

15. You have a young patient with true divergence excess. The exophoria at far is 10 prism diopters, and he is orthophoric at near. Symptoms are blurred vision and discomfort when looking at television and far distances. An optical therapy approach to consider is prescribing _____ spectacle lenses.
   a. base-in prisms in single vision
   b. base-out prisms in single vision
   c. minus-addition in single vision
   d. plus addition bifocals

16. You have a patient with divergence excess who is wearing bifocals. The type of vergence training taking place during reading and other near work is considered to be _____, and the goal of this vision therapy is to increase the _____ ranges.
   a. jump, base-in
   b. sliding, base-out
   c. tromboning, base-in
   d. isometric, base-out

17. You have a patient with divergence excess in which the far deviation is 20 prism diopters and the near deviation is 10 exophoric. You prescribe plus and minus 2.00 diopter lens rock using a flipper holder, and a vectographic target at 40 centimeters with a suppression check in which a small circle encompasses a vertical line seen only by the right eye and a line directly below it that is seen only by the left eye. This, in effect, is a fixation disparity target. When the −2.00D lenses are interjected, the top line for the right eye would probably be:
   a. suppressed
   b. vertically aligned with the bottom line
   c. seen to the left of the bottom line
   d. seen to the right of the bottom line

18. You have a 12-year-old patient who is 2 prism diopters exophoric at 6 meters and 12 prism diopters exophoric at 40 centimeters. He is symptomatic with complaints of blurring and fatigue with near work, especially with prolonged reading. This seems to be a case of _____ with the diagnosis being _____.
    a. divergence excess, complete
    b. divergence excess, incomplete
    c. convergence insufficiency, complete
    d. convergence insufficiency, incomplete

19. You prescribe chiastopic fusion training for a patient with exophoria at near and far. The targets are separated 90 millimeters apart. When viewed from a distance of 30 centimeters, the fusional convergence demand is _____ prism diopters, and when viewed from a distance of 3 meters, the fusional convergence demand is _____ prism diopters.
    a. 3, 30
    b. 15, 30
    c. 30, 3
    d. 30, 15

20. You have a 10-year-old patient with intermittent exotropia of 20 prism diopters at 6 meters and 40 centimeters. You prescribe chiastopic fusion as one of several home training techniques. Generally, patients master the technique at near more _____ than at far, although the magnitude of the demand on fusional convergence is _____ at far if the separation of the two targets is kept constant.
    a. slowly, less
    b. quickly, more
    c. slowly, more
    d. quickly, less

21. Generally accepted norms for base-in to blur, break, and recover at a testing distance of 40 centimeters are _____, and for base-out to blur, break, and recover, they are _____.
    a. 6/10/5, 15/19/8
    b. 12/20/11, 15/19/8
    c. 12/20/11, 6/10/5
    d. 6/10/5, 12/20/11

22. A young patient is brought to you because his parents say that he complains of blurring of vision when reading, yet he passed the Snellen chart test at school and has 20/20 in each eye. Your examination reveals convergence insufficiency. The most likely reason for the complaint of blurring is because the convergence demand is beyond the patient's limit of positive _____, and positive _____ takes over to avoid diplopia.
   a. total vergence, fusional vergence
   b. accommodative convergence, fusional vergence
   c. fusional vergence, accommodative convergence
   d. total vergence, accommodative convergence

23. You have a patient who has intermittent esotropia of 15 prism diopters at 6 meters and 5 prism diopters at 40 centimeters. The AC/A ratio is _____, and this vergence anomaly would be classified as:
   a. 10/1, convergence excess
   b. 5/1, divergence excess
   c. 2/1, divergence insufficiency
   d. 1/1, basic esodeviation

24. You have an esophoric patient with divergence insufficiency. An approach to therapy for which you should be cautious is:
   a. base-in fusional training
   b. pencil push-aways
   c. base-out relieving prisms for general wear
   d. base-out Fresnel prisms in the upper segment of the spectacle lenses

25. When determining the AC/A ratio with the cover test and prisms, the "cross-link" between accommodation and convergence is _____ as opposed to the gradient method in which the "cross-link" is _____, and convergence may stimulate accommodation because of the _____ ratio.
   a. open, closed, CA/C
   b. closed, open, AC/A
   c. open, closed, AC/A
   d. closed, open, CA/C

Answers

1. b. More leeway is given to accommodative lag than to excess. A lag of small amount is normally found in most patients. A lag less than 0.75 may be ideal. An excess of accommodation (lead of accommodation) may indicate spasm, pseudomyopia, or other causes.

2. c. As with most testing procedures of accommodative and vergence functions, ametropia of each eye should be corrected before testing. The push-up procedure is performed with the other eye occluded. The test is done monocularly to avoid vergence being a factor in the measurement.

3. a. Accommodative facility with binocular testing, especially with suppression monitoring, is less than with monocular testing. Monocular speed in not hampered by co-existing vergence demands. Adequate monocular accommodative facility would be 10 to 13 cycles per minute. Unless suppression is monitored, the patient can perform almost as though being monocular if there is suppression of an eye.

4. b. The exodeviation increased by 5 prism diopters as a result of the +1.00D lens addition, thus a 5/1 ratio. It is important to point out that the accommodative response is variable and not always the same as the accommodative stimulus. The gradient method may be inconsistent as regards the response ratio. Nevertheless, the stimulus gradient procedure is useful in clinical practice.

5. b. The absolute convergence represented by the phoria line would be to the left of the demand line and parallel to it because the slope (6/1) is the same as the demand line. When the exodeviation becomes greater at near, the slope becomes less steep.

6. d. The esodeviation at near due to the high AC/A ratio and the patient being symptomatic indicates an esodeviation problem at near, which are characteristic of a convergence excess binocular anomaly.

7. c. A plus-addition add would theoretically reduce the near esodeviation. Single vision lenses would not be satisfactory because of blurring of distant vision.

8. c. With the high AC/A ratio of 10/1, a +1.50D addition would
        theoretically have an effect of 15 prism diopters, resulting in
        exophoria of 3 prism diopters $(12 - 15 = -3)$. This would not
        be a desirable outcome as it pertains to vision therapy in a case
        of convergence excess in which fusional divergence is to be
        improved.

9. a. An important rule is to progress from easy to difficult vision
        training techniques. A patient can easily fuse the pencil tip with
        the pushup technique. The aperture-rule trainer is dissociative,
        and the double aperture is used for fusional divergence demands.
        This is sometimes difficult for patients initially trying to fuse
        with clear single vision. Orthopic (uncrossed) fusion in the open
        environment is the most difficult technique for many patients
        to master.

10. b. In cases of convergence excess, fusional divergence demands
        are increasingly introduced as the target is moved closer to the
        patient. This is because of the high AC/A ratio making the
        patient's esodeviation increase as the viewing distance decreases.
        The patient must use fusional divergence to see the target
        singly.

11. d. The absolute convergence can be calculated using the formula:
        prism diopters = IPD $(100/x + 2.7)$ where x represents the
        7-centimeter distance from the spectacle plane to the point of
        bifixation $[6(100/7 + 2.7) = 62]$.

12. a. In cases of convergence insufficiency, the patient cannot rely solely
        on accommodative convergence when trying to meet the demand
        for bifixation. Fusional convergence must contribute in order to
        meet the demand to maintain singleness as the target moves closer
        and the exodeviation becomes larger.

13. a. Relative convergence is the fusional convergence measured and
        specified with reference to the position of the eyes corresponding
        to the normal fusional demand for the given testing distance.
        Positive fusional vergence ("positive" meaning convergence and
        "negative" meaning divergence) includes the compensatory
        vergence needed to meet the orthophoric position, and it also
        includes relative convergence. Chiastopic fusion presents the
        patient with base-out demands.

14. b. This value can be determined with simple trigonometry; however, a convenient and useful clinical way is to use the "decimeter rule," which gives the number of millimeters it takes to equal 1 prism diopter at that viewing distance. In this example, the fixation distance is 4 decimeters. It takes 40 mm to equal 10 prism diopters. This rule can be applied to similarly split targets, such as with cards in a Brewster stereoscope, vectograms, or chiastopic fusion in free space.

15. d. Assume the patient has an AC/A ratio of 10/1. A +1.00D addition lens, for example, would theoretically result in an exodeviation at near of 10 prism diopters. The rationale in vision therapy is to make the near and far exodeviations approximately the same. In this way, the patient will be using the same fusional effort and near and far, and when looking from near to far there will not be a dramatic change as it would be otherwise without the bifocals.

16. d. The goal is to increase base-out fusion ranges, without blur. Jump vergence means that bifixation is quickly changed from one distance to another with accommodative stimulus changing likewise. Tromboning is similar to jump vergence except that the target to be bifixated is moved slowly from one distance to another. Sliding vergence means that base-in and base-out demands are introduced beyond that of the orthophoric position while the accommodative stimulus remains the same, because the target distance remains the same. Isometric vergence means that the accommodative stimulus stays the same while the convergence stays at the orthophoric demand position.

17. d. This patient has a 10/1 AC/A ratio, theoretically creating an accommodative-convergence response of 20 prism diopters; thus, an esodeviation of 10 prism diopters would result. An esophoric fixation disparity is likely with homonymous projection so that the right eye would see the top line displaced to the right of the bottom line.

18. d. Although much of the classification of vergence anomalies, convergence insufficiency in this case, is based on the relationship between the far and near deviations, there are other findings necessary for a complete diagnosis. Findings such as the nearpoint of convergence, fusional convergence, and facility of vergence are important.

19. c. A clinically simple way to know what convergence demands are put on the patient at these distances is to divide the 90-millimeter separation by the decimeter viewing distance. For near, it would be 90/3 = 30 prism diopters base-out; at far, it would be 90/30 = 3 prism diopters base-out.

20. d. There are several reasons fusion is easier at near than far, such as (1) stereopsis provides "glue" to hold fusion at near; (2) proximal convergence may help; and (3) image sizes of near targets are larger than at far using the same targets, tactile and kinesthetic feedback help at near, especially to hold attention. Note that the demand on fusional convergence, as well as absolute convergence, is mathematically less at far than at near.

21. b. It not surprising that nearpoint divergence values are similar to the convergence values, because it is within established norms, and in the general population, a range of orthophoria to 6 prism diopters of exophoria is considered normal.

22. c. First blurring is perceived when the limit of positive fusional vergence, with base-out demand, is reached. After that point, accommodative convergence comes into play and a lead of accommodation causes blurring. The positive total convergence (combination of fusional and accommodative convergence) limit is reached when diplopia begins. An explanation in lay terms of this effect is helpful in explaining to patients why binocular anomalies can cause blurred vision, notwithstanding 20/20 (6/6) vision when tested monocularly.

23. c. The AC/A ratio is low [6 + 0.4(5 − 15) = 2/1]. The low AC/A ratio in this case of esodeviation is the reason the near deviation is much less than the far deviation, which is characteristic of divergence insufficiency.

24. c. Base-out relieving prisms may be good for the greater esodeviation at far but bad for the near esodeviation, which is much less. Too much base-out prism power can make the patient "optically exophoric" at near. The patient, therefore, would be training fusional convergence when reading and doing near work. The objective in therapy in this case is to improve fusional divergence with base-in training. Pencil push-aways can be used to work on fusional divergence because the esodeviation becomes greater as the target distance increases. As a short-term optical relief, Fresnel base-out prisms can be regionally placed at the top of the spectacle lenses for distant viewing while the patient can look through the bottom portion of the spectacle lenses for near work.

25. a. When an eye is occluded, as with the cover test, this opens the cross-linking, feedback-loop in the relationship between accommodation and convergence. In natural binocular seeing conditions, however, individuals have a closed "loop" in that there is on-going interaction with feedback between accommodation and convergence. Convergence can stimulate accommodation [convergence-accommodation/convergence (CA/C)], just as accommodation can stimulate convergence (accommodative-convergence/accommodation [AC/A]). While application of the AC/A ratio is clinically useful, the clinician needs to keep these interactions in mind and realize that the AC/A ratio is not always linear and the slope can change at times, e.g., influence of pharmaceutical agents and vision training. These interactions also have an effect on tonicity of accommodation and convergence resulting in adaptations, such as vergence ("prism") adaptation, which can often be helpful in vision therapy for binocular anomalies.

CHAPTER 33

Refractive Correction Applications

Nancy Peterson-Klein, James R. Miller,
Robert Buckingham, Michael P. Keating,
Bruce Morgan, Philip E. Walling

1. For a high-powered spherical spectacle prescription, a laboratory returns a lens with the correct spherocylindrical parameters but a base curve that differs significantly from the corrected curve lens base curves specified for that power. For this lens, the main effect of the monochromatic aberrations of this lens will be:
   a. the appearance to the patient of colored fringes around bright lights and/or at high contrast borders
   b. an incorrect lensometer power reading through the optical center
   c. decreased visual acuity when the patient looks off-axis (up, down, left, or right) through the lens
   d. decreased light transmittance through the lens

2. A patient desires a pair of spectacle lenses with excellent impact resistance but does not want polycarbonate. Which of the following lenses materials will best meet the patient's specifications?
   a. ophthalmic crown glass
   b. flint glass
   c. CR-39
   d. trivex
   e. 1.60 index plastic

3. A hyperopic patient wants a lightweight spectacle correction with the thinnest possible center. Which of the following spectacle lens choices will work best?
   a. aspheric CR-39
   b. aspheric 1.60 index plastic
   c. spherical CR-39
   d. spherical 1.60 index plastic
   e. polycarbonate with a 1-mm center thickness

4. An aphakic patient has just put on his first spectacle correction since the surgery. The spectacle-corrected aphakic complains that doors about 10 feet away appear to bend inward to the point that he is unsure whether he will fit through the door. The optical aberration responsible for this effect is:
    a. spherical aberration
    b. curvature of field
    c. radial astigmatism
    d. distortion
    e. coma

5. A patient wants the lightest-weight lenses that she can get. Based on density only, which of the following lens materials would work best for this patient?
    a. polycarbonate
    b. CR-39 plastic
    c. ophthalmic crown glass
    d. 1.60 index plastic
    e. 1.90 index glass

6. Two different CR-39 spectacle lenses of the same fairly large diameter are made for a 9.00-D myope. Each lens is centered and has a round shape and a 2.0-mm center thickness. Lens A has a +2.00-D front surface and lens B has a +7.00-D front surface. What is the relative relationship of the edge thickness of these two lenses?
    a. both lenses A and B have zero edge thickness (i.e., knife edge)
    b. lenses A and B have equal edge thickness that is greater than zero
    c. lens B has a thicker edge than lens A
    d. lens A has at thicker edge than lens B

7. What are the advantages of an FT-28 flat top bifocal over an RD-28 round seg bifocal?
    a. less jump and a wider horizontal field of view near the top of the seg
    b. less jump and a narrower horizontal field of view near the top of the seg
    c. more jump and a wider horizontal field of view near the top of the seg
    d. more jump and a narrower horizontal field of view near the top of the seg

8. Which parameter is characteristic of a spectacle lens material that gives the smallest amount of chromatic aberration for a plus lens?
    a. low index of refraction
    b. high index of refraction
    c. low Abbe value
    d. high Abbe value

9. Which patient is most likely to complain about an overly restricted field of view?
   a. spectacle-corrected hyperope
   b. contact lens-corrected hyperope
   c. spectacle-corrected myope
   d. contact lens-corrected myope

10. A patient returns to your office complaining about a new spectacle lens. The spherocylindrical and prism parameters of the lens are acceptable, and you do not see any problems with the clarity of the lens. Of the following, what is the MOST likely source of the problem with the lens?
    a. stria
    b. centering error
    c. waves
    d. elliptical error

11. Which spectacle lens would MOST benefit from an antireflection coating?
    a. low index
    b. high index
    c. high density
    d. low density

12. Which of the following visible light transmittances would work BEST for sunglasses for a young to middle-aged person?
    a. 5%
    b. 15%
    c. 40%
    d. 80%

13. A spectacle-corrected presbyopic high hyperope complains that she has to look too far vertically down to read at near through her bifocal segment. For the same seg height, which of the following bifocals would minimize this effect?
    a. flat-top 28
    b. executive (Franklin style)
    c. round 22
    d. round 38

14. A patient has a spectacle RX of OD –3.00 D and OS –7.00 D with a +2.00 D add OU. The patient selects flattop bifocals. The near reference point (NRP) is 10 mm below the distance reference point (DRP). This patient returns complaining of double vision when looking through the add. How much reverse slab (i.e., base down) prism and on which lens will alleviate the problem?
    a. 3△ on the right lens
    b. 3△ on the left lens
    c. 4△ on the right lens
    d. 4△ on the left lens
    e. 7△ on the right lens

15. A spectacle-corrected presbyopic emmetrope complains that while reading a newspaper she often loses her place when her line of sight passes from the distance portion to the near portion of her bifocal. Which of the following spectacle lenses will work BEST to minimize this problem?
    a. progressive add lens with a long corridor
    b. bifocal with a round 22 seg
    c. bifocal with a flat-top 28 seg
    d. bifocal with a flat-top 35 seg
    e. single vision lens with distance power

16. A patient selects a frame that is accurately marked 52 □ 20. The patient's Rx is −5.50 −1.25 × 180 OU, and the patient's PD (symmetric) is 64 mm. What decentration relative to the geometric center is needed for each lens to avoid any unwanted horizontal prism in the Rx?
    a. 2 mm in
    b. 3 mm in
    c. 4 mm in
    d. 5 mm in
    e. none of the above since the required decentration is out

17. A spectacle-corrected presbyopic hyperope looking at an intermediate distance complains that his field of view is too narrow horizontally. Which of the following lenses would work BEST for solving this problem?
    a. short corridor progressive add lens
    b. long corridor progressive add lens
    c. single vision lens with near power
    d. round trifocal 6 × 22
    e. flat-top trifocal 8 × 35

18. A lens clock (or lens measure) reads +8.00 D on the front surface of a 1.70 index spherical plastic lens and −6.00 D on the back surface of the lens. The base curve of this lens is:
    a. −6.00 D
    b. +8.00 D
    c. plus with a magnitude that is greater than 8.00 D
    d. minus with a magnitude that is greater than 6.00 D
    e. plus with a magnitude that is less than 8.00 D

19. Typically, which of the following progressive add lenses would have the least unwanted astigmatism in the lower nasal and temporal parts of the lens?
    a. short corridor and horizontally wide clear near vision area
    b. short corridor and horizontally narrow clear near vision area
    c. long corridor and horizontally wide clear near vision area
    d. long corridor and horizontally narrow clear near vision area

20. When measuring the spherocylindrical parameters of a single vision lens with a lensometer, the cylinder axis wheel reads 180; one set of lines is clear when the power wheel reads +3.00 D; and the perpendicular set of lines is clear when the power wheel reads −2.00 D. The minus cylinder power in the single vision lens is:
    a. −1.00 D
    b. −2.00 D
    c. −3.00 D
    d. −5.00 D
    e. −6.00 D

21. The seg height of a bifocal is the distance from the seg top to the:
    a. seg bottom
    b. optical center of the seg
    c. distance reference point
    d. geometric center of the lens
    e. bottom boxing line

22. The procedure to accurately determine the add on a high plus spherical plastic RD-22 bifocal lens is:
    a. measure both the near power and distance power with the back surface of the lens against the lensometer stop, and subtract the two readings
    b. measure both the near power and distance power with the front surface of the lens against the lensometer stop, and subtract the two readings
    c. measure the near power with the front surface of the lens against the lensometer stop, measure the distance power with the back surface of the lens against the lensometer stop, and subtract the two readings
    d. measure the near power with the front surface of the lens against the lensometer stop and record that number
    e. measure the near power with the back surface of the lens against the lensometer stop and record that number

23. When checking the prism power in a spherical distance vision spectacle correction for a young myope, what part of the spherical single vision lens needs to be placed directly over the lensometer stop?
    a. geometric center
    b. optical center
    c. boxing center
    d. near reference point
    e. distance reference point

24. A patient's OS spectacle Rx is $-3.00 -1.25 \times 180$ combined with 2.50^Δ BU prism. When the lens is properly placed against the lensometer stop, how is the intersection of the center sphere lines with the center cylinder lines positioned relative to the center of the reticle circles?
    a. the intersection point is vertically above the center of the reticle circles
    b. the intersection point is vertically below the center of the reticle circles
    c. the intersection point is displaced nasally from the center of the reticle circles
    d. the intersection point is displaced temporally from the center of the reticle circles
    e. the intersection point lies exactly in the center of the reticle circles

25. A spherocylindrical spectacle correction for a compound hyperopic astigmat with a large amount of astigmatism is correctly positioned against a lensometer stop. To directly measure the minus cylinder power and axis of the spectacle lens (i.e., without any need for transposition) with a lensometer, the user next needs to:
    a. start with the power wheel at high plus and turn it toward lower plus (or eventually higher minus) until the cylinder lines come clear first, the sphere lines comes clear second; subtract reading one from reading two for the power, and then read the axis wheel
    b. start with the power wheel at high plus and turn it toward lower plus (or eventually higher minus) until the sphere lines come clear first, the cylinder lines comes clear second; subtract reading one from reading two for the power, and then read the axis wheel
    c. start with the power wheel at high minus and turn it toward lower minus (or eventually higher plus) until the cylinder lines come clear first, record that reading, and then read the axis wheel
    d. start with the power wheel at high minus and turn it toward lower minus (or eventually higher plus) until the sphere lines come clear first, record that reading, and then read the axis wheel

26. A 24-year-old patient has a new glasses prescription of a +4.00 −3.75 × 180 OU and complains of objects appearing oblong. Which of the following procedures would NOT relieve this problem?
    a. decrease the sphere power
    b. reduce the amount of cylinder
    c. constant wearing of glasses for 2 weeks
    d. a gradual increase in the power of the cylinder

27. Which of the following prescriptions has a mixed astigmatism?
    a. plano +1.00 × 090
    b. −1.00 +2.00 × 090
    c. −2.00 +2.00 × 180
    d. +1.00 +1.00 × 045

28. How many refracting surfaces does a fused D-25 bifocal have in the reading portion of the lens?
    a. one
    b. two
    c. three
    d. four

29. What modification should be made in the adjustment of a spectacle frame with a −15.00 D lens when the wearer complains that distant objects appear blurred?
   a. lengthen the temples to move the spectacles away from the eyes
   b. spread the adjustable nose pads to bring the lenses closer to the eyes
   c. adjust the nose pads so that the patient is looking through the optical centers
   d. adjusting the spectacle frame will not have an effect on the patient's blurred vision

30. After a car accident, a patient has a refraction of OD −5.00 DS add +2.50 DS and OS −1.50 DS add +2.50 DS. The patient does not appear to be troubled by aniseikonia. However, when reading through her new executive bifocal glasses, she complains of vertical diplopia. An examination reveals that the patient reads 0.6 cm below the optical center of the reading section. Which of the following options would NOT reduce the prismatic effect?
   a. increase the "A" size on the glasses
   b. use contact lenses rather than glasses
   c. lower the optical centers in the reading section
   d. use two pairs of glasses, one for distance and one for near

31. A patient complains that when she is walking, the ground appears distorted while she wears her new glasses. She states this never happened with her old glasses. Her old glasses are +5.25 DS OU. You verify her new glasses and they are also a +5.25 DS OU. Which of the following is the least likely cause of the problem?
   a. uncorrected residual astigmatism
   b. different panoscopic tilt between the spectacles
   c. different base curves between the old and new glasses
   d. patient looks through different parts of the lenses between the old and new spectacles

32. A patient complains of the thickness of his lenses. When advising the patient, which of the following lens materials would produce the thinnest lenses?
   a. trivex
   b. HI-index
   c. polycarbonate
   d. aspheric mid-index

33. You dispense to a patient new glasses that incorporate lenticular lenses. What problem associated with lenticular lenses should the doctor discuss with the patient at the time of dispensing?
    a. blurred vision
    b. temple length
    c. small field of vision
    d. minification of objects

34. You are dispensing new spectacles to a 15-year-old girl who has never worn glasses before. Her prescription is OD plano −1.50 × 103 and OS −0.25 −1.75 × 077. Which of the following is the most important information to mention to her?
    a. round objects now appearing oval
    b. objects appearing smaller than normal
    c. blurred vision through the spectacles especially at night
    d. the ground being closer to her when looking through her bifocal

35. A common cause of contact lens problems in computer users is related to which of the following factors?
    a. UV radiation from the screen
    b. reduced blink rate
    c. reduced tear production
    d. IR radiation from the screen

36. What technique is available to measure the K-readings of an advanced keratoconic patient whose readings are off the scale?
    a. add a +1.25 D trial lens in front of the keratometer objective
    b. add a +2.75 D trial lens in front of the keratometer objective
    c. K-readings are not possible in a patient with keratoconus
    d. add a −1.25 D trial lens in front of the keratometer objective

37. A well-fitting soft lens will exhibit all of the following EXCEPT:
    a. corneal coverage in all positions of gaze
    b. smooth return on push-up test
    c. 1-mm post blink movement
    d. edge alignment to the conjunctiva

38. Symptoms of initial discomfort when inserting a soft trial lens are NOT commonly related to:
    a. excessive edge stand-off from the conjunctiva
    b. differences between tear pH and the pH of the storage solutions
    c. insufficient lens movement
    d. excessive lens movement caused by a loose lens and reflex tearing

39. Which of the following will have the greatest impact on tightening a contact lens fit?
    a. flatten base curve radius (BCR), increase overall diameter (OAD)
    b. steepen BCR, decrease OAD
    c. flatten BCR, decrease OAD
    d. steepen BCR, increase OAD

40. A patient requesting GP lenses has K-readings of 7.58 mm at 180 and 7.42 mm at 90. Which spherical back surface GP lens with a standard OAD/OZD of 9.4/7.8 mm should result in an alignment fluorescein pattern?
    a. 7.63 mm
    b. 7.54 mm
    c. 7.42 mm
    d. 7.38 mm

41. With which of the following prescriptions will a spherical GP lens NOT provide satisfactory vision?
    a. K's: 42.00 at 090 × 43.00 at 180   Rx: −2.00 − 1.00 × 090
    b. K's: 44.50 at 180 × 45.50 at 090   Rx: −1.00 −2.50 × 180
    c. K's: 43.50 at 180 × 45.50 at 090   Rx: −3.00 −2.00 × 180
    d. K's: 44.50 at 180 × 44.50 at 090   Rx: −2.50 DS DS

42. An unlikely cause of poor vision in a GP lens wearer would be:
    a. excessive edge lift
    b. poor wetting
    c. lens flexure
    d. lens warpage

43. Which of the following lenses should be chosen to achieve the same optical correction as a lens with a BCR of 7.58 mm and a power of +2.00 D?
    a. 7.50 mm, +2.25 D
    b. 7.67 mm, +1.50 D
    c. 7.50 mm, +2.50 D
    d. 7.67 mm, +2.50 D

44. A spectacle refraction is found to be −5.00 −2.50 × 010 at vertex distance 10 mm. What soft lens toric power would you initially trial?
    a. −4.75 −2.50 × 010
    b. −5.25 −2.00 × 010
    c. −4.75 −2.25 × 010
    d. −4.25 −2.75 × 010

45. An ocular refraction is found to be –4.00 –1.75 × 170. A trial soft toric contact lens with an Rx of –3.75 –1.75 × 180 placed on the eye rotates counterclockwise by 10 degrees. What lens prescription would you order to compensate for this rotation?
    a. –4.00 –1.75 × 180
    b. –4.00 –1.75 × 160
    c. –4.00 –1.75 × 170
    d. –4.00 –1.75 × 080

46. A patient corrected to 20/20 OD and OS is given a distance target and a +2.00 D lens is held alternatively over each eye. The patient reports that the image is clearest when the lens is held before the right eye. This blur test would indicate:
    a. the patient is left eye dominant
    b. no strong dominance is present
    c. the patient is right eye dominant
    d. the patient is left handed

47. When fitting a simultaneous vision bifocal contact lens, which of the following statements is FALSE?
    a. objective vision measurement alone is not a good predictor of success
    b. overrefraction using a phoropter is preferred
    c. 0.25 D adjustments can have a significant effect on visual performance
    d. lens centration is important
    e. overrefraction should be performed in normal room illumination

48. When fitting segmented alternating vision bifocal contact lenses, the segment top position during primary gaze should be approximately:
    a. in line with the upper pupil margin
    b. bisecting the pupil horizontally
    c. in line with the lower pupil margin
    d. midway between lower pupil margin and inferior limbus

49. Which of the following factors is most likely to influence a decision to choose a GP aspheric multifocal design versus a GP alternating bifocal design?
    a. lower lid 2 mm below the limbus
    b. add greater than +2.00 D
    c. large pupils
    d. critical near vision demand

50. Which of the following clinical observations is more likely to result in patient symptoms?
    a. vascularization
    b. microcysts
    c. low-grade GPC
    d. infiltrate (no overlying epithelial defect)
    e. diffuse epithelial staining resulting from toxic reaction

51. Which of the following solution properties has the least effect on initial comfort?
    a. low pH
    b. viscosity
    c. tonicity
    d. preservative concentration
    e. high pH

52. Which of the following conditions is less likely to be observed with silicone hydrogel materials compared with hydrogel lenses?
    a. SEAL lesions
    b. "mucin balls"
    c. corneal edema
    d. infiltrates
    e. CLARE

53. GP contact lenses are useful in therapeutic lens fitting because they:
    a. are more comfortable
    b. allow greater tear exchange
    c. are fitted with smaller total diameters
    d. form a liquid tear lens and smooth refracting surface
    e. have higher oxygen transmissibility

54. During follow-up of an extended wear bandage lens fit, which of the following may NOT be necessary?
    a. assessment of lens fit
    b. visual acuity measurement
    c. slit lamp examination
    d. assessment of tissue healing
    e. lens removal

55. A first-year medical resident wears her daily wear soft lenses for 18 to 20 hours a day. You diagnose corneal hypoxia. What would be the BEST option for this patient?
    a. decrease wearing time to 8 hours a day
    b. prescribe a low water content lens to be worn extended wear
    c. prescribe a thick, high water content lens
    d. consider a silicone hydrogel for daily wear

56. A patient has 39.50 @ 180; 40.00 @ 090 K readings OU and a spectacle Rx of OD −2.00 DS and OS −1.75 −0.50 × 180. What base curve and power would you choose for an initial soft lens fitting?
   a. medium BC OU, −2.00 D OD, −1.75 D OS
   b. flattest BC OU, −2.25 D OD, e−1.75 D OS
   c. medium BC OU, −1.75 D OD, −2.00 D OS
   d. flattest BC OU, −2.00 D OU

57. A contact lens patient with corneal edema will often present with the following:
   a. halos or hazy vision
   b. generalized injection
   c. diffuse stipple staining of the cornea
   d. increased vision toward the end of the day

58. Giant papillary conjunctivitis often presents with the following:
   a. unilateral presentation
   b. initial itching worse upon lens insertion
   c. excessive lens movement
   d. watery discharge

59. If water content is increased in an HEMA lens, which of the following is true?
   a. oxygen permeability will always increase
   b. oxygen transmission will always increase
   c. resistance to deposits will always increase
   d. contact lens dehydration is always decreased
   e. oxygen transmission will always decrease

60. The optimal movement of a soft contact lens in straight ahead gaze is:
   a. 1.5 to 2.0 mm
   b. 0.5 to 1.0 mm
   c. 0.5 mm
   d. >2.0 mm

61. If a contact lens patient presents with reduced visual acuity, the first follow-up question should be:
   a. could your lenses be switched?
   b. are you having any discharge?
   c. is the reduced vision with contact lenses only?
   d. have you had any trauma to the eye?

62. If a contact lens patient is taking an oral antihistamine or is on oral contraceptives, which of the following symptoms is more likely to occur?
     a. photophobia
     b. itching
     c. dryness or gritty feeling
     d. euphoria

63. If striae are detected in a soft contact lens patient, the following treatment is indicated:
     a. refit with a lens of higher Dk/t value
     b. tighten the fit
     c. prescribe frequent lubricants
     d. change solution regimen

64. The linear measurement of a contact lens representing the base curve is the:
     a. blend
     b. overall diameter
     c. optic zone
     d. front optic zone

65. For two different curves to have the same sag, the flatter curve must:
     a. have the same size chord diameter as the steeper
     b. have a smaller chord diameter
     c. have a larger chord diameter
     d. neither a, b, nor c

66. A bifocal contact lens that allows light rays from various distances to focus on the retina at the same time is called a(an):
     a. alternating vision bifocal
     b. segmented bifocal
     c. concentric bifocal
     d. simultaneous vision bifocal

67. If you decrease the peripheral curve width of a GP lens and steepen the peripheral curve radius, the Z-value (edge clearance) will:
     a. increase
     b. decrease
     c. stay the same
     d. depend on lens material

68. Which of the following is used in contact lens solutions primarily because it is a chelating agent?
     a. BAK
     b. EDTA
     c. thimerosal
     d. chlorhexidine

69. If an ultrathin hydrogel lens shows very little movement, you should:
    a. immediately refit to flatter base curve
    b. try push-up test
    c. have the patient massage their lid
    d. immediately refit to a larger diameter lens

70. The main concern over the use of tap water with contact lenses is:
    a. rust rings on the lens
    b. burning upon insertion
    c. acanthamoeba
    d. iritis

Answers

1. c. The monochromatic aberrations of radial astigmatism (astigmatic error) and curvature of field (power error) will result in some blurring of the retinal image when the person looks off-axis.

2. d. Trivex and polycarbonate are the two lens materials that far exceed the others in terms of impact resistance.

3. b. Higher index lenses are thinner. Asphericity also makes the lens thinner.

4. d. This is pincushion distortion.

5. a. Polycarbonate has the lowest density of these choices. Trivex was not a choice, but it has an even lower density than polycarbonate. The lower density of polycarbonate will offset the slightly smaller lens thickness of 1.60 plastic. The 1.90 index glass will be thinner, but glass has a much higher density than plastic materials.

6. c. For a higher-powered lens, steeper lenses are thicker than flatter lenses. For a lens of lower powers, the difference may not be significant.

7. a. The FT-28 is horizontally wider near the top of the seg and so has a wider horizontal field of view. Relative to the RD-28, the FT-28 bifocal has a segment optical center that is closer to the top of the seg and thus has a smaller prismatic jump.

8. d. The chromatic aberration in diopters equals the lens power divided by the Abbe value. So a lens material with a higher Abbe value results in a smaller amount of chromatic aberration.

9. a. A contact lens moves with the eye and so restricts the field of view. The spectacle lens diameter constitutes a field of view restriction (a field stop). A minus correction minifies the image and gives a larger field of view, and a plus correction (hyperope) magnifies the image and gives a smaller field of view.

10. c. In any plastic lens material, but particularly high index plastics, heat buildup during the surfacing/edging/coating process can cause localized waves on the surface of the lens. While waves are small enough to not be apparent when looking at the lens, they can cause an apparent localized distortion when viewing through the lens and can cause a patient to reject a lens.

11. b. A high index lens reflects more light (has a decreased transmittance) and therefore would most benefit from an antireflection coating.

12. b. A visible light transmittance in the general range of 10% to 20% would work well. Most sunglasses fall into approximately a 12% to 16% transmittance zone. The light transmittance of the crystalline lens decreases as a person ages, so an older person's sunglasses may need a higher transmittance.

13. d. The round 38 seg has the vertically lowest seg optical center. So it has the most base down prism near the top of the seg and would be best at minimizing the effect.

14. c. At the near reference point (NRP), the distance powers give 3^Δ BD on the right lens and 7^Δ BD on the left lens (Prentice's rule). This is a vertical prism imbalance (VPI) of 4^Δ. Reverse slab prism is base down, so 4^Δ reverse slab on the right lens makes a total of 7^Δ BD on the right lens and eliminates the VPI.

15. a. A progressive add lens has no vertical prismatic jump and will be best at minimizing this problem.

16. c. The DBC (or frame PD) is 72 mm and the patient's PD (symmetric) is 64 mm. 72 minus 64 is 8 mm, and 8 divided by 2 is 4 mm decentration in.

17. e. The flat-top 8×35 has the horizontally widest intermediate seg width.

18. b. For this lens, the base curve by definition is the lens clock (lens measure or lens gauge) reading, +8.00 D, on the front surface of the lens. Note: this is not the true power of the front surface. The true power would be plus and greater than 8.00 D.

19. d. Typically spreading out the dioptric power transition minimizes the amount of the amount of unwanted astigmatism. The long corridor and horizontally narrow clear near vision area provide for the largest spread in the power transition.

20. d. The readings are the dioptric powers in the principal meridians and the cylinder power is the difference (–3 D minus +2 D), which is –5.00 D.

21. e. Geometric lens parameters are specified by the boxing system.

22. b. This is a high plus lens, so there can be significant changes in light vergence across the interior of the lens. The add comes from the difference in surface powers at the front of the lens, and for an accurate measurement of that, the front surface of the lens needs to be against the lensometer stop.

23. e. This is a single vision lens question and not a progressive add lens question. For a single vision lens, the only place on this lens that has a prism power numerically equal to the prescribed prism is at the distance reference point.

24. a. When directly looking through BU prism, the object appears to be deviated down (or toward the apex). However, the keplerian telescope on the lensometer inverts the image, and hence the lensometer target displacement will be up relative to the center of the reticle circles.

25. b. To have the correct axis reading on the axis wheel, the sphere lines needs to be focused first. Then the subtraction in b gives the minus cylinder power.

26. a. The problem is due to a change in the astigmatism. Decreasing the sphere power will not have an effect on the complaints.

27. b. Mixed astigmatism is the condition where one meridian focuses in front of the retina and the other meridian focuses beyond the retina.

28. c. A fused bifocal will have three refracting surfaces: the anterior surface of the fused button, the posterior surface of the fused button, and the posterior surface of the lens.

29. b. For minus lenses, bringing the lenses closer to the patient will increase the overall power.

30. a. Increasing the "A" size on the glasses will have no effect on vertical prism. The other three options would decrease the prismatic effect.

31. a. Uncorrected astigmatism would have the same effect on both pair of spectacles. However, panoscopic tilt changes, base curve changes, and viewing angle can affect the patient's perceptions.

32. b. HI-index material would produce the thinnest lenses available.

33. c. Lenticular lenses cause a smaller field of view due to the design of the lens.

34. a. Due to the new astigmatic correction, the patient will now notice that round objects appear oval or square objects appear as rectangles. At the dispensing, the doctor should advise the patient of this phenomenon.

35. b. It has been found that the blink rate reduces during computer use (by as much as 60%), potentially leading to inferior corneal desiccation and dry eye symptoms. A blinking regimen and tear supplements should be given.

36. a. A +1.25 D lens may be used in conjunction with the instrument and the use of a conversion table for excessively steep corneas. Minus lenses are rarely needed for an excessively flat cornea.

37. c. Movement of a soft lens plays little part in corneal oxygenation, and movement of 1 mm on blinking is excessive and would likely increase patient awareness of the lens. Good corneal coverage is essential to avoid desiccation of the cornea. Smooth return on push-up and edge alignment are both characteristics of a good fit.

38. c. It is common for a very tight lens to initially feel very comfortable, due to a decrease in mechanical irritation of adjoining tissue.

39. d. Both steepening the BCR and increasing the OAD will serve to increase the sag of the lens and tighten the fit.

40. a. As the cornea is aspheric and flattens away from the center, in most corneas selecting a base curve for a GP lens that is slightly flatter than "K" (the flatter corneal meridian; in this case 7.58 mm) should result in an alignment lens-to-cornea fitting relationship. Therefore, a 7.63 mm base curve (i.e., 0.25 D flatter than K) should result in this pattern. The other selections should all result in apical clearance.

41. b. There is 2.50 D of cylinder in the spectacle refraction, whereas the K readings indicate that only 1.00 D of this is corneal. The remaining 1.50 D is likely to be lenticular, and this would remain uncorrected if a spherical GP lens were fitted.

42. a. Excessive edge clearance would decrease comfort, but it would not directly decrease vision.

43. d. The lens is flatter by 0.50 D, which results in a −0.50 D tear lens. Therefore, in this case, it is necessary to add +0.50 D to the lens power (SAMFAP: Steep Add Minus, Flat Add Plus).

44.   c.   The reduced sphere and cylinder power reflect the reduction in minus lens power needed *in each meridian* the closer one is to the cornea.

45.   b.   Counterclockwise indicates a rotation to the right when looking at the patient. Applying LARS (Left Add Right Subtract) to the *spectacle* axis results in an axis of 160. By specifying an axis of 160, the counterclockwise rotation of 10 degrees will leave the lens oriented at the 170 axis required.

46.   a.   A successful monovision patient is able to somewhat suppress the blurred image. By significantly blurring with +2.00 D either eye, the patient will report clearer or more comfortable vision when the fog is presented before the nondominant eye. This method has been shown to be more accurate than the preferred sighting method.

47.   c.   The simultaneous lens design relies upon a change in the refractive power of the lens from the center to the periphery and therefore is highly pupil dependent. Testing should be done with loose lenses in normal room illumination to best simulate normal wearing conditions. Use of a phoropter will decrease light entering the eye and tend to cause mydriasis. Lens centration is important for optimal optical performance at distance and near.

48.   c.   By placing the segment top in line with the lower pupil margin in the primary gaze position, the lens will translate up upon downgaze and the near segment will be over the pupil.

49.   a.   Ideally, a lower lid positioned at or near the limbus will provide the most stability and improve translation upon downgaze for an alternating design. Typically, an alternating design is better suited for more critical near demand and higher adds, which can be directly incorporated into the segment versus relying on the optics of asphericity. Alternating designs are also not as pupil dependent as aspheric designs.

50.   e.   Although there is always great subjective variation between patients in the reporting of any symptom, there is unlikely to be any symptom reported with neovascularization, microcysts, or infiltrates without staining. Low-grade GPC, where papillae have yet to be established significantly, is unlikely to result in either discomfort or blurring from the tear film. Because of the distribution of corneal nerves, there is an associated discomfort with epithelial compromise and the diffuse stain found as a response to a toxic reaction typically presents with reports of discomfort after a period of wear.

51.   b.   As viscosity is linked less to the presence of ions in solution than the other options, it will have less effect on initial comfort.

52.   c.   Corneal edema is less likely with silicone hydrogels as they have excellent oxygen transmission to help avoid this.

53.   d.   The GP lens provides a smooth refracting surface over the top of the liquid tear lens and significantly improves the visual potential of any cornea that has been compromised. This would be the case with, for example, keratoconus, epithelial dystrophies, and iatrogenic or traumatic corneal scarring.

54.   e.   Lens removal may not be necessary providing there is an adequate view of the relevant ocular structures and there is no indication for changing or improving the lens.

55.   d.   Although decreasing the wearing time would decrease the likelihood of hypoxia, it would greatly affect the lifestyle of the patient. A silicone hydrogel lens worn on a daily wear basis would likely give the patient the desired wearing schedule and significantly reduce hypoxia due to its high Dk value. Extended wear would only add to the hypoxia and a thick lens would again decrease oxygen transmission.

56.   d.   K readings indicate a flat corneal topography and spherical equivalent power of OS equals –2.00 D.

57.   a.   The swelling of the cornea induces diffraction of light and decreased corneal transparency, inducing halos around lights and hazy vision, particularly later in the day. Injection and staining are not directly associated with corneal edema.

58.   c.   The papillae on the upper tarsal conjunctiva often interact with the lens by pulling it excessively upward with the blink. GPC is almost always bilateral, produces a ropy/mucous discharge, and incites itching mainly after lens removal.

59.   a.   Increased water content in an HEMA lens will always increase the Dk, but transmissibility is dependent on the lens thickness as well, and therefore a higher water content may be offset by an increase in thickness. Deposit resistance usually decreases with an increase in water content and dehydration increases.

60.   b.   Movement greater than 1.0 mm has no physiologic benefit and only serves to increase lens awareness.

61. c. Asking this question will reduce your differential diagnoses by half by narrowing the problem to either a lens-related or an eye-related issue.

62. c. Antihistamines and oral contraceptives both contribute to aqueous tear deficiency and may lead to dry eye symptoms in contact lens wearers.

63. a. Striae are one of the first indicators of corneal edema, and therefore increased oxygen transmission is necessary. Tightening a lens fit will tend to inhibit tear exchange and decrease oxygen transmission, and the other options would have no effect.

64. c. Overall diameter includes the peripheral curve widths, blend indicates the transition between peripheral curves, and the front optic zone is unrelated to the base curve.

65. c. Sag will always decrease with flatter lenses if the chord diameter (essentially the optic zone diameter) remains constant. For sag to remain constant, the chord length (OZD) must lengthen for a flatter lens.

66. d. Alternating and segmented bifocal contact lenses have two distinct powers, one for distance and one for near, that are focused on the retina independently. Some concentric designs are alternating, prism ballasted designs as well.

67. b. Edge clearance decreases when either PC is narrowed or steepened and more so if both are used. Increased edge lift is achieved by widening and/or flattening the PC, and edge lift is independent of lens material.

68. b. EDTA (ethylenediaminetetraacetate) is used in conjunction with preservatives to enhance their antibacterial action, particularly against *Pseudomonas*. The other choices are true preservatives.

69. b. Many current hydrogel lenses have low profile edges that interact very little with the lids. A positive push-up test using the lower lid showing fluid movement over the limbus and smooth return to centration is deemed adequate. If the push-up test is negative, a flatter base curve would be indicated.

70. c. *Acanthamoeba* infection is directly related to the use of tap water and is a high risk for serious vision loss. Rust rings on a hydrogel lens are an indication that tap water is being used, and the patient should be educated appropriately.

Part 3 Recommended Reading

Amos J, ed: *Diagnosis and management in vision care.* Boston, 1987, Butterworth-Heinemann.

Benjamin WJ, Borish IM: *Borish's clinical refraction.* Philadelphia, 1998, Saunders.

Burian HM: *Burian-von Noorden's binocular vision and ocular motility: theory and management of strabismus,* St Louis, 1980, Mosby.

Caloroso EE, Rouse MW: *Clinical management of strabismus,* Boston, 1993, Butterworth-Heinemann.

Carlson NB, Kurtz D: *Clinical procedures for ocular examination*, ed 3, New York, 2004, McGraw-Hill.

Evans BJW: *Pickwell's vision anomalies: investigation and treatment,* ed 4, Oxford, 2002, Butterworth-Heinemann.

Garzia R: *Vision and reading,* St Louis, 1996, Mosby.

Gasson A, Morris J: *The contact lens manual: a practical guide to fitting,* Oxford, UK, 2003, Butterworth-Heinemann.

Griffin JR, Grisham JD: *Binocular anomalies: diagnosis and vision therapy*, ed 4, Boston, 2002, Butterworth-Heinemann.

Grosvenor T: *Primary care optometry*, ed 3, Boston, 1996, Butterworth-Heinemann.

Hofstetter HW, Griffin JG, Berman MS, Everson RW: *Dictionary of visual science and related clinical terms,* ed 5, Boston, 2000, Butterworth-Heinemann.

Jalie M: *Ophthalmic lenses & dispensing,* Edinburgh, 2003, Butterworth-Heinemann.

Kaufman PL, Alm A: *Adler's physiology of the eye: clinical application*, St Louis, 2003, Mosby.

Keating MP: *Geometric, physical, and visual optics,* Boston, 2002, Butterworth-Heinemann.

Lens A: *Ocular anatomy and physiology,* Chicago, 1999, SLACK.

Maino DM: *Diagnosis and management of special populations,* St. Louis, 1995, Mosby.

Michaels DD: *Visual optics and refraction: a clinical approach,* St Louis, 1985, Mosby.

Moore BD: *Eye care for infants and young children,* Boston, 1997, Butterworth-Heinemann.

Moore P: *Clinical pediatric optometry,* Boston, 1993, Butterworth-Heinemann.

Rutstein R, Daum K: *Anomalies of binocular vision,* St Louis, 1998, Mosby.

Scheiman M, Wick B: *Clinical management of binocular vision*, ed 2, Philadelphia, 2002, Lippincott Williams & Wilkins.

Scheiman R: *Optometric management of learning related vision problems,* ed 2, St Louis, 2006, Mosby.

Von Noorden GK, Campos EC: *Binocular vision and ocular motility: theory and management of strabismus,* ed 6, St Louis, 2002, Mosby.

Weissberg EM, et al: *Essentials of clinical binocular vision,* St Louis, 2004, Butterworth-Heinemann.

Werner DL, Press LJ: *Clinical pearls in refractive care,* Boston, 2002, Butterworth-Heinemann.

PART 4

Perceptual Conditions

CHAPTER 34

Anomalies of Child Development

Elise B. Ciner, Gale Orlansky

1. A 4-year-old boy is brought in due to concerns that he has a color deficiency. He is able to name all of the brightly colored blocks you present to him. This means that:
   a. he does not have an acquired color deficiency
   b. he has a receptive language problem
   c. his expressive language skills are not well developed
   d. he may have an inherited color deficiency

2. The Denver Development Screening Test is composed of the following four areas:
   a. personal/social; cognitive; visual motor; language
   b. cognitive; visual perception; language; gross motor
   c. language; visual perception; gross motor; eye-hand coordination
   d. personal/social; fine motor/adaptive; language; gross motor

3. A test to assess a 3-year-old child's visual motor skills would be:
   a. Beery test of visual motor integration
   b. Gardner test of reversal frequency
   c. circus puzzle
   d. walking rail

4. An optometrist should be concerned by a child who does not appear to know left and right on themselves by age:
   a. 3 years
   b. 4 years
   c. 6 years
   d. 8 years
   e. 10 years

5. A test of auditory visual integration that can be used for children beginning in kindergarten is the:
   a. Birch Belmont test
   b. DEM
   c. TVPS
   d. standing angels

6. The "Token Test" can be used to assess what aspect of perception at what age?
   a. reversals beginning at age 3
   b. reversals beginning at age 5
   c. receptive language beginning at age 3
   d. receptive language beginning at age 5

7. A 3-year-old presents to your office for an evaluation due to concerns that she is not coloring the way that are other children in her day care. A good test to administer to gain an understanding of her visual motor skills relative to the chief complaint would be:
   a. Beery test of visual motor integration
   b. Winterhaven copy forms test
   c. grooved pegboard
   d. DTLA test of visual motor speed and precision

8. A child in third grade is brought in because he is unable to write neatly in school. What two tests would be most appropriate to administer?
   a. DEM and TVPS
   b. TVPS and Wold sentence copy
   c. Gardner recognition and TVPS
   d. TVAS and Wold sentence copy
   e. DEM and Piaget left-right awareness

9. In school-age children with learning disabilities, the probability of an associated visual perceptual disorder is approximately:
   a. 1 in 5
   b. 2 in 5
   c. 3 in 5
   d. 4 in 5
   e. 5 in 5

10. An 8-year-old child presents to your office with no specific visual complaints but a history of poor grades since kindergarten. If you were to find a visual problem, it would most likely be which of the following?
    a. moderate myopia
    b. convergence insufficiency
    c. visual processing disorder
    d. mild astigmatism

11. A 5-year-old boy was referred for an eye examination by his kindergarten teacher because he was not able to keep up with the other children in the class. Your evaluation shows the following vision problem that could be contributing to the chief complaint:
    a. divergence excess strabismus
    b. 1 diopter of hyperopia in each eye
    c. 1 diopter of astigmatism in each eye
    d. 40th percentile performance on the test of auditory analysis
    e. 20th percentile performance on the Beery test of visual motor integration

12. One of the most common chromosomal deficits that occur in 1 in 1000 live births is:
    a. trisomy 13
    b. trisomy 18
    c. trisomy 21
    d. disomy 15
    e. disomy 18

13. Short palpebral fissures (the length of the eye opening), a flat midface, an indistinct or flat philtrum, a thin upper vermillion, and a short nose are common features in what condition?
    a. trisomy 18
    b. athetoid cerebral palsy
    c. fetal alcohol syndrome
    d. Down syndrome
    e. Little's disease

14. Children with cerebral palsy:
    a. have symptoms that worsen with time
    b. have associated mental retardation in almost all cases
    c. have a condition that cannot be inherited
    d. rarely have strabismus
    e. most commonly have the athetoid type

15. One of the first identified genetic etiologies of learning disabilities is:
    a. Down syndrome
    b. cerebral palsy
    c. fetal alcohol syndrome
    d. fragile X syndrome
    e. dyslexia

16. Mental retardation in fragile X syndrome is manifested more frequently in:
    a. males
    b. females
    c. infants
    d. no difference between males or females

17. The prevalence of cerebral palsy in the United States is approximately 1 in:
    a. 10,000
    b. 100,000
    c. 500,000
    d. 1,000,000
    e. 5,000,000

18. A 10-year-old girl with spastic cerebral palsy presents to your office for an eye examination. You are most likely to see what group of clinical findings?
    a. significant refractive error, ptosis, accommodative insufficiency
    b. color vision deficit, strabismus, accommodative insufficiency
    c. peripheral retinal degeneration, strabismus, Brushfield spots
    d. sixth nerve palsy, retinal degeneration, color vision deficit
    e. strabismus, significant refractive error, accommodative insufficiency

19. Which of the following conditions is associated with congenital heart defects, good socialization skills, and increased susceptibility to leukemia?
    a. pervasive developmental disorder
    b. autism
    c. trisomy 21
    d. neurofibromatosis

20. A high myopic refractive error is typically seen in which of the following developmental disabilities?
    a. albinism
    b. Treacher Collins syndrome
    c. autism
    d. Stickler's syndrome

21. A 6-year-old child comes into your office for an eye examination. In the course of taking a history, you determine that she is having trouble learning to read. Your eye examination does not show any significant vision problem, and a visual perceptual examination is also negative. In talking with the parents after your evaluation, the most appropriate recommendation you can make would be a referral for:
    a. an auditory processing examination
    b. a psychoeducational examination
    c. a reading test
    d. an electrodiagnostic evaluation

22. Which of the following is NOT a symptom of ADHD?
    a. fidgeting
    b. poor organizational skills
    c. problems with handwriting
    d. focusing difficulties

23. A child is seated for a perceptual examination. During testing, he is looking around the examination room and tapping his pencil on the table, and he lacks interest with the test set before him. What test would best support your diagnosis of this child's style of learning?
    a. Wold sentence copy test
    b. matching familiar figures test
    c. Detroit test of motor speed and precision
    d. TVPS-R test-visual memory
    e. Beery test of visual motor integration

24. A 10-year-old girl has a full-scale IQ of 105. The child's performance IQ is 15 points below the verbal IQ. The results of the visual perceptual evaluation are below average. What can the optometrist do to help this child?
    a. the child has above average intelligence, so no intervention is needed
    b. the child is in need of eyeglasses to improve her performance IQ
    c. the performance subtest scaled scores range between 5 and 13, which is within one standard deviation from the mean; therefore, no intervention is needed
    d. the optometrist should note that there is a significant difference between the verbal and performance IQ and the visual perceptual disorder should be addressed with vision therapy

25. Which one of the following is NOT a test of visual motor integration skills?
    a. Winterhaven copy forms
    b. grooved pegboard
    c. test of visual analysis skills
    d. Beery-Buktenica developmental test
    e. all of the above tests are tests of visual motor integration

26. A 4-year-old child comes in for a routine vision examination. Your examination is essentially normal, except that the child cannot match pictures for visual acuity testing and is not able to understand many of the instructions during the examination. You perform Forced Choice Preferential Looking in order to obtain a visual acuity of 20/20 in each eye. You should consider:
    a. seeing this child again in 1 year for a routine vision evaluation
    b. refer this child to a pediatric ophthalmologist
    c. refer this child to a neurologist
    d. refer this child to a developmental pediatrician
    e. refer this child to an occupational therapist

27. Results of an IQ test can best aid the optometrist in deciding whether there is a vision-related learning disability by:
    a. asking the child if he or she enjoyed the testing
    b. comparing the results of the performance IQ and the verbal IQ
    c. looking at the full-scale IQ score to see if it is below average
    d. comparing the results of the reading assessment with the child's grade in school
    e. asking the child if he or she enjoyed the picture arrangement subtest

28. The WISC has recently been revised to include:
    a. an assessment of processing speed
    b. a test of foreign language comprehension
    c. an assessment of cultural bias
    d. an evaluation of hyperactivity

29. The most frequent form of inherited mental retardation is:
    a. cerebral palsy
    b. fragile X syndrome
    c. Turner's syndrome
    d. trisomy 12
    e. Marfan's syndrome

30. A 7-year-old girl reports difficulty completing paper and pencil tasks required for her second-grade class. Your evaluation indicates the child has a visual-motor deficit that requires vision therapy. The rest of her examination is unremarkable. What additional evaluation by her school can you recommend to help her overcome her academic difficulty?
    a. referral to the school nurse
    b. referral to a physical therapist at her school
    c. referral to an occupational therapist at her school
    d. referral to the speech and language therapist at her school
    e. No referral is necessary

31. When evaluating a 9-year-old child who is having academic difficulties, a good test of intersensory integration is:
    a. Gardner test of reversal frequency–matching subtest
    b. test of auditory analysis skills
    c. Birch Belmont test
    d. TVPS subtest of visual memory
    e. TVPS subtest of visual closure

32. A child with a dyseidetic classification of dyslexia would have the following IQ profile:
    a. low verbal, low performance
    b. low verbal, high performance
    c. high verbal, high performance
    d. high verbal, low performance

33. Which of the following are examples of sequential visual processing?
    a. TVPS closure; Beery VMI
    b. TVPS form constancy; grooved pegboard
    c. Birch Belmont; Wold sentence copy
    d. Gardner reversal matching; standing angels

34. A child with sloppy handwriting or drawing skills, poor spacing, and inability to stay on lines who has difficulty producing answers on paper and has difficulty completing written work in the allotted time would most likely be diagnosed with what type of visual processing deficit?
    a. bilateral integration
    b. visual memory
    c. auditory-visual integration
    d. visual-motor integration
    e. directionality

35. A 7-year-old patient is able to identify right and left on his own body (lateral awareness) but is unable to correctly identify the direction of letters and numbers on a page (directionality). The treatment for this patient would NOT include which one of the following tests?
    a. Kirschner arrows
    b. stickman figures
    c. road map
    d. rotating pegboard

Answers

1. d. The results say nothing about the presence or absence of an acquired color deficiency. He is able to say and name all of the colors, ruling out b and c. Even though he can distinguish the brightly colored blocks, he could still have a mild inherited color deficiency.

2. d. The Denver developmental screening test is widely used by optometrists to gain an overall developmental level of a child. It is a tool that is easily used to help make appropriate referrals to pediatricians or therapists. It can also be helpful to determine what types of optometric tests the child might respond to and helps "warm" the child up to the testing environment.

3. c. The Beery test is generally useful for children aged 4 years and older. The Gardner is a test for reversals in older children, and the walking rail is used for gross motor assessment and therapy. The circus puzzle is a good test to assess visual perception, visually guided behavior, and visual motor skills in 3-year-olds.

4. c. Children should know left and right on themselves by age 6 years.

5. a. The Birch Belmont test of auditory integration assesses this area. The DEM (developmental eye movement test) is a test of eye movements, the TVPS (test of visual perceptual skills) evaluates nonmotor visual perception, and standing angels is a gross motor test of bilateral integration.

6. c. The "token test" assesses receptive language function and the ability to follow directions in a visual setting. Normative data are available beginning at age 3 years (through age 12.5 years).

7. b. Although all four of these are tests of visual motor integration, only the Winterhaven copy forms is appropriate for her age level and for her chief complaint.

8. d. The TVAS (test of visual analysis skills) and the Wold sentence copy are the only tests listed that both measure visual motor integration (although slightly differently). The Wold sentence copy requires the child to attempt to copy a sentence in 1 minute, whereas the TVAS evaluates form perception with visual motor feedback by connecting dots on a map to form a specific pattern.

9. b. Of children diagnosed with a learning disability, approximately 1 in 5 has a pure visual perceptual basis for their learning disability, and another 1 in 5 has a visual perceptual deficit mixed with other factors (total = 2 in 5).

10. c. Visual efficiency disorders (a, b, and d) generally do not affect a child in the younger grades when the nearpoint demand is low and the print is large. Children with visual processing delays typically have difficulty learning how to read, which occurs in the early grades; therefore, answer c is the most likely possibility.

11. e. Answers a through c generally do not contribute to learning difficulties in the early grades. The 40th percentile is within the average range of performance on the TAAS. While the 20th percentile on the Beery is in the low average range of performance, it is the most likely condition listed here that is contributing to this child's difficulties.

12. c. Trisomy 21, also known as Down syndrome, is one of the most common chromosomal deficits present in children who survive to birth (50% of fetuses spontaneously abort).

13. c. These are all characteristics of fetal alcohol syndrome. The philtrim is the ridge under the nose. The vermillion is the lip.

14. c. Children with cerebral palsy have a condition that does not worsen with time. A third of these children have normal intelligence. Strabismus is common (15% to 69%). The spastic type (60% to 80% of cases) is far more common than the athetoid type (10% to 20% of cases).

15. d. Fragile X syndrome is one of the first causes of learning disabilities that can be directly traced to a genetic defect.

16. a. Four out of every five males have IQ in mental impairment, whereas only one third of females have IQ in the mental retardation range. This is because females have two X chromosomes. Females with fragile X have one normal FMR1 gene (fragile X gene) and one mutated FMR1 gene in most of their cells. In contrast, males only have one X chromosome, resulting in a significant increase in signs and symptoms of fragile X syndrome.

17. c. The prevalence of CP in the United States has remained the same or risen slightly due to better early care and survival of premature infants.

18. e. The prevalence rates of strabismus (15% to 69%), accommodative insufficiency (85% to 95%), and refractive errors (40% to 76%) are higher than the other conditions, which are either not seen in cerebral palsy (i.e., Brushfield spots) or have a low prevalence (color vision in girls).

19. c. Trisomy 21 is the only choice that has all of the listed conditions associated with it.

20. d. Albinism typically presents with hyperopia and astigmatism. Treacher Collins syndrome is associated with astigmatism, and autism is not associated with any specific refractive error. Only Stickler's syndrome is commonly associated with myopia.

21. b. A psychoeducational evaluation would provide the parent with an overall assessment of their child's intellectual abilities and academic skills. Following this evaluation, appropriate further referrals to an audiologist or reading specialist can be made. There is no indication for electrodiagnostic testing.

22. c. Handwriting is not considered a symptom of ADHD; it is indicative of a visual motor problem.

23. b. Although observation of a child's attention to a task could be assessed with any of the above tests, the matching familiar figures test was specifically developed to assess visual attention and concentration.

24. d. The child's full scale IQ does fall within the average range: 90 to 109. However, in this situation where the visual perceptual tests results are below average and the performance IQ is below the verbal IQ by 12 or more points, this is considered a significant difference. This usually indicates that the visual perceptual disorder is problematic for the child in question.

25. e. All of these tests are tests of visual motor integration. The Beery is the most widely used test due to its reliability and it is normed to a greater age range than the others.

26. d. This child's visual evaluation is essentially normal, except that the child appears to be exhibiting some delays in speech, perceptual, and cognitive skills. The most appropriate action from the list given is referral to a developmental pediatrician. (Assessment of visual perceptual skills would also have been appropriate if this were a choice.)

27. b. By comparing the results of the performance and verbal IQ, the optometrist can gain an understanding of whether the child might have a learning-related vision problem. Children with high verbal and low performance IQ are more likely to have a visual problem contributing to their learning disability.

28. a. The newly revised WISC now includes assessments of verbal comprehension, perceptual organization, freedom from distractibility, and processing speed.

29. b. Fragile X syndrome is now thought to be the most common form of inherited mental retardation.

30. c. The occupational therapist (OT) at her school can provide an evaluation and possible therapy to complement the vision therapy she will receive. The OT can observe the activities required in the classroom and work directly with her to improve her skills.

31. c. The Birch Belmont test of auditory visual integration evaluates a child's ability to equate a temporally distributed auditory stimulus to a spatially distributed visual response. It is, therefore, a test of intersensory integration. The other choices are primarily assessing nonmotor visual perceptual skills (choices a, d, and e), and the TAAS is testing auditory analysis skills.

32. d. The dyseidetic and dysphonetic classification is another way to categorize dyslexia. Dysphonetic individuals have a primary difficulty with symbol-sound integration, whereas those classified as dyseidetic have difficulty with visual processing skills. Therefore, an individual with a dyseidetic classification would have a high verbal and low performance IQ, whereas an individual with a dysphonetic classification would be more likely to have a low verbal and higher performance IQ.

33. c. The Birch Belmont and Wold sentence copy tests both have a component that takes place over time. The Birch Belmont requires the child to remember a temporal sequence of sounds and to relate it to a visual display, while the Wold sentence copy requires the child to sequentially copy a sentence over the period of 1 minute. The grooved pegboard could also be considered as having a sequential component to it, but the TVPS does not as the task is one of simultaneous processing where all the pieces are in front of the child and the child has to synthesize an answer on each page. None of the other tests has a sequential processing component.

34.   d.   While this child may have other difficulties as well, the symptoms are most directly correlated with a deficit in visual-motor integration.

35.   d.   The rotating pegboard is more commonly used during ocular motor training and not for directional skills. The Kirschner arrows, stickman figures, and road map require the child to have an internal awareness of right and left on himself so he can be able to organize his external space.

CHAPTER 35

Anomalies of the Aging Adult

Vasudevan Lakshminarayanan

1. Approximately what percentage of patients with diabetes also show ocular involvement at the time of diagnosis of their disease?
   a. 20% to 40%
   b. 10% to 20%
   c. 40% to 60%
   d. 60% to 80%

2. A sign of preretinopathy in diabetic patients is the presence of:
   a. dot and blot hemorrhages
   b. dilated tortuous veins
   c. macular edema
   d. cotton wool patches

3. Which of the following is NOT associated with secondary aging?
   a. cardiovascular disease
   b. cerebrovascular disease
   c. presbyopia and cataract
   d. diabetes

4. Color vision changes in the aging patient are usually due to:
   a. yellowing of crystalline lens
   b. physiologic and pathologic changes in macula
   c. alterations of photoreceptor absorption spectra
   d. a, b, and c
   e. a and b

5. When refracting the elderly patient, it is important to take into account the fact that:
   a. there is a shift from with-the-rule to against-the-rule astigmatism
   b. there is a shift from against-the-rule to with-the-rule astigmatism
   c. the aging crystalline lens shows increasing dioptric power in the horizontal meridian relative to the vertical
   d. the aging crystalline lens shows increasing dioptric power in the vertical meridian relative to the horizontal
   e. a and c

6. Elderly individuals, when performing versional eye movements:
   a. show a decreased gain (increased lag)
   b. show a greater number of saccades
   c. are more restricted in vertical movements than in movements in other directions
   d. a, b, and c

7. According to Sheedy and Saladin, in regard to functional vergence and age:
   a. positive fusional vergence decreases with age
   b. negative fusional vergence does not decrease with age
   c. positive fusional vergence increases with age
   d. a and b
   e. b and c

8. Variability in visual performance between individuals as a function of age:
   a. increases for virtually all tasks
   b. increases for certain tasks
   c. does not change for all tasks

9. Senile miosis could be due to:
   a. atrophy of dilator muscle fibers
   b. increased rigidity of blood vessels
   c. a and b
   d. variation in pigment density

10. It is found that the depth of the anterior chamber decreases from about 3.6 mm at age 20 to above 3.0 mm at age 70, because of growth of the lens. This will consequently:
    a. increase the refractive power of the eye, making it relatively more myopic
    b. increase the refractive power of the eye, making it relatively more hyperopic
    c. decrease the refractive power of the eye, making it relatively more myopic
    d. decrease the refractive power of the eye, making it relatively more hyperopic

11. The amount of light reaching the retina of a normal 60-year-old is
     about _____ that reaching the retina of a normal 20-year-old.
     a. one half
     b. two thirds
     c. one third
     d. three fourths

12. An elderly observer will see an increase in _____, which will
     tend to reduce contrast.
     a. fluorescence
     b. scatter
     c. retinal illuminance
     d. a and b

13. When performing a subjective refraction on an aged patient, it might
     be necessary for you, the optometrist, to use a 0.5-D or 0.62-D instead
     of the usual 0.37-D crossed cylinder in the determination of
     astigmatism. This is because:
     a. of the reduced retinal illuminance
     b. the diameter of retinal blue circles is small
     c. of the smaller depth of focus
     d. of the larger depth of focus

14. Thyrotoxicosis can occur with muscle palsy and the general signs
     could include (choose **incorrect** answer):
     a. Van Graefe's sign
     b. exophthalmos
     c. vertical diplopia
     d. frequent blinking

15. With age tear production diminishes. This can lead to (choose **correct**
     answer):
     a. desiccation
     b. scarring
     c. dry eye syndrome
     d. dellen

16. Aging changes in the cornea could include:
     a. stippling of Bowman's membrane
     b. Hassall-Henle bodies
     c. arcus senilis
     d. a, b, and c

17. Ischemic optic neuropathy has a peak incidence in the _____ decade of life.
    a. sixth
    b. fifth
    c. fourth
    d. seventh

18. Disability glare is a major problem in the elderly because of:
    a. increased sensitivity to light
    b. increased intraocular light scatter
    c. pupillary miosis
    d. variation of the Stiles Crawford effect with age

19. In the elderly, there could be reduced oxygen transmission to the cornea. This could be due to:
    a. degeneration of subepithelial tissue
    b. pterygia
    c. lid ptosis
    d. a, b, and c

20. Some common problems with aphakic spectacle correction are:
    a. pin cushion distortion
    b. restricted visual field
    c. altered depth perception
    d. a, b, and c

21. With age, the ERG B-wave amplitude:
    a. increases with increasing age
    b. is not significantly correlated with age
    c. decreases with increasing age
    d. is directly proportional to illumination level

22. The clinician should be careful about interpreting fluorescein angiograms of elderly patients because:
    a. elderly patients typically have a slow filling rate for the retinal optic disc and peripapillary choroidal vessels
    b. elderly patients typically have a fast filling rate for the retinal optic disc and peripapillary choroidal vessels
    c. elderly patients have too many fluoregens in the retina, producing fluorescence "noise" in the image

23. When fitting contact lenses in the elderly, the optometrist should be careful because patients might not complain of pain with an ill-fitting lens. This is because:
    a. corneal sensitivity to touch increases with age
    b. corneal sensitivity to touch decreases with age
    c. there is a change in corneal thickness
    d. there is an increase in against-the-rule astigmatism

24. With age, which of the following is NOT true?
    a. the lens capsule thickness increases
    b. elastic modules of the lens capsule decrease
    c. zonular contractility increases
    d. permeability of lens capsule increases

25. Which of the following is NOT a general risk factor for cataracts?
    a. hypertension
    b. steroid use
    c. elevated estrogen level
    d. high antioxidant index

26. Which of the following does NOT change or become negated by normal aging?
    a. Stiles Crawford effect of the first kind
    b. spherical aberration
    c. longitudinal chromatic aberration
    d. a, b, and c

27. When refracting the elderly (choose **incorrect** answer), the optometrist must take into account:
    a. increase in reaction time
    b. decrements in hearing
    c. smaller JNDs (just noticeable differences)
    d. longer testing time

28. Reading disability in Parkinson's disease is related to:
    a. failure of eyes to converge
    b. inability to perform normal saccadic eye movements
    c. inability to move the eyes into downgaze
    d. a, b, and c

29. Visual disorders in Alzheimer's disease include:
    a. visual agnosia
    b. spatial agnosia
    c. visual spatial disturbance
    d. a, b, and c

30. When fitting an elderly patient with spectacles, do NOT:
    a. choose a large frame
    b. use high index plastic lenses
    c. use silicone nose pads
    d. use a small frame

31. Color coding such as those used on medication labels may be potentially confusing to an elderly person because:
    a. there is less contrast as a result of papillary miosis
    b. because of increased absorption, especially at the lower wavelengths, leading to a tritan type color vision deficiency
    c. because of increased absorption, especially at the longer wavelengths, leading to a tritan-type color vision deficiency
    d. because of increased absorption, especially at the middle wavelengths, leading to a deutan-type color deficiency

32. Possible postreceptor mechanism for age-related loss in visual function could be:
    a. reduced receptor pooling
    b. decreased levels of retinal neurotransmitters
    c. decreased response amplitude of neurons
    d. cortical cell loss
    e. a, b, c, and d

33. In many standard clinical tests, it is critical that the elderly be encouraged to continue to read a letter chart or to respond to the stimulus because:
    a. the elderly tend to adopt a stringent, more conservative response criterion
    b. the elderly will not respond unless they are "rewarded"
    c. it will enable the elderly to guess and hence have a lower threshold (or better visual function)
    d. the elderly need extremely strong orders from the authority figure, namely the clinician
    e. a and c

34. If you measure a dark adaptation curve in an elderly subject, you will find that:
    a. the thresholds during the entire time course of dark adaptation are similar to those of younger observers
    b. the thresholds are elevated during the entire course of dark adaptation compared with younger observers
    c. the cone portion of the dark adaptation curve is similar to that of younger observers but the rod portion thresholds are elevated
    d. the thresholds in the cone portion of the dark adaptation curve are elevated, but rod portion thresholds are similar to those of younger observers

35. In the elderly, spatial contrast sensitivity shows a:
    a. general decline at all spatial frequencies
    b. decline at low and intermediate frequencies
    c. decline at intermediate and high spatial frequencies
    d. decline at high and low spatial frequencies

Answers

1. a. Diabetes is the most important systemic disease leading to blindness; the majority of diabetic blind patients are middle-aged or elderly. Because diabetes has a peak age of onset that coincides with the onset of presbyopia, optometrists can recognize this disease in its early stages.

2. b. Preretinopathy is difficult to identify because the definitive signs of dilated veins and tortuosity are common in normal subjects and in eyes of patients having other vascular diseases. Diabetic retinopathy is generally classified as preretinopathy, simple or background retinopathy, a transition stage, and proliferative retinopathy.

3. c. Secondary aging is defined as aging processes that have been accelerated because of otherwise uncontrollable or preventable circumstances. On the other hand, presbyopia and cataract are anatomic/physiologic changes associated with the "normal" aging process.

4. e. Because of increased scatter and absorption, especially in the short wavelengths, as well as changes in the macula, color vision defects will occur in the aged patients. In general, defects tend to be tritanopic with a reduction in discrimination in the blue and blue-green regions of the spectrum.

5. e. There is a change in corneal curvature leading to an increase in against-the-rule-astigmatism. The power of the cornea increases with age, especially in the horizontal meridian.

6. d. It is found that even at relatively slow target movements, older adults show decreased gain and an increased number of saccades. The range of voluntary eye movements becomes limited.

7. d. Sheedy and Saladin report that the decrease in positive fusional vergence is far greater than the increase in near exophoria. (See Sheedy JE, Saladin JJ: Exophoria at near in presbyopia, *Am J Optom Physiol Opt* 52:474-481, 1975.)

8. a. There is considerable variability, and this increases with age for nearly all visual performance tasks. This makes it difficult to assess "what is normal" and "below normal" performance.

9. c. Senile miosis is thought to be due to both of these reasons and is one of the most significant changes in the aging eye. The difference in the diameter of the pupil between light and dark adapted eyes becomes smaller.

10. a. The contraction of the anterior chamber is due to lens growth and due to its forward displacement. It is estimated that the anterior chamber decreases by about 0.1 mm every year after the age of 20 years. This corresponds to an increase in power of the eye of approximately 0.5 D/decade of life. (See, for example, pp 69-70 of Weale RA: *The senescence of human vision,* New York, 1992, Oxford University Press.)

11. c. This can be easily calculated by noting that the amount of light falling on the retina is directly proportional to the square of the pupillary radius.

12. d. As the lens grows, it accumulates two fluorogens, one of which is activated by light of short wavelength and fluoresces at a longer wavelength. There is also an increase in the mass of certain protein molecules of high molecular weight, which tend to accumulate near the nucleus of the lens. These molecules act as scatterers.

13. b. As a result of miosis, not only is retinal illumination reduced, but the diameter of blur circles are also small. On subjective refraction, changes in lens power will not change blue circle diameters as much as similar change in eyes with larger pupils, hence the need for higher powers.

14. b. Thyrotoxicosis can occur with muscle palsy but without the exophthalmos. Patients usually find it difficult to elevate their eyes, because more than one muscle is involved. A contracture of the inferior rectus is common. Clinical signs could include retraction of the upper lid, infrequent blinking, conjunctival injection, etc.

15. c. Excess tear evaporation could play a significant role in dry eye syndrome. Keratitis sicca is an aqueous deficiency and is different from Sjögren syndrome, which is characterized by dry eyes.

16. d. Age-related changes of the cornea could include stippling of Bowman's membrane, destruction of Bowman's membrane near the limbus (white limbus girdle), excrescences on Descemet's membrane (Hassall-Henle bodies), and arcus senilis.

17. a. This is primarily a disease of the elderly, and the peak incidence occurs in the sixth decade. (See page 140 of Rosenbloom AA, Morgan MW: *Vision and aging,* ed 2, Boston, 1993, Butterworth Heinemann.)

18. b. Because of aging changes in the lens, there is greater light scatter. Stiles Crawford effect is relatively invariant with eye.

19. c. With age, there is a reduction in muscle tone, amount of orbital fat, and elasticity.

20. d. Optically the difficulties arise from magnification, incorrect pantoscopic tilt, improper vertex distance, pincushion distortion, improper face form tilt, and ring scotoma ("jack in the box" phenomenon) as well as restricted visual field. These give rise to altered depth perception, hand-eye coordination difficulties, maintenance of spectacle vertex distance for optimal acuity, binocularity, restricted visual field, and cosmesis.

21. c. The ERG B-wave amplitude decreases with increasing age, especially after age 50. This decrease is even more evident if the intensity of the stimulus is increased. The latency, however, does not decrease (if the ocular media is clear).

22. a. Because of the slow filling in rate, it can be interpreted as hypofluorescence. Appropriate age-adjusted norms should be used.

23. b. Corneal sensitivity to touch decreases with age. The threshold for touch almost doubles between the ages of 10 and 80, increasing rapidly after the age of 40. As a result, the elderly might not be aware of corneal lesions without being aware of subjective symptoms. (See Millodot M: Influence of age on the sensitivity of the cornea, *Invest Ophthalmol Vis Sci* 16:240-272, 1977.)

24. c. With age, the lens axial thickness increases by about 28% at age 70 over that at the age of 20. The other changes, such as decrease in elastic module and increased lens permeability, are also well documented. However, with age, there is a decrease in zonular contractility and hence a reduction in the ability to accommodate. (See, for example, pp 63-67 of Weale RA: *The senescence of human vision,* New York, 1992, Oxford University Press.)

25. d. The causes of cataract can be congenital, toxic, metabolic, traumatic, or senescent. It appears as though high antioxidant levels are not etiologic factors in cataract formation.

26. d.   The Stiles Crawford effect of the first kind is one of visual
          functions invariant with age. Other invariant visual functions
          include certain types of hyperacuity stimuli (two-dot Vernier
          acuity) and the positions of the neutral points (unique hues) and
          the white point.

27. c.   It appears as though the elderly have a larger JND between
          incremental selections. This will necessitate the use of larger
          incremental changes (i.e., use of 0.50 DS instead of 0.25 DS).

28. d.   Parkinson's disease patients may have eye movement problems and
          complain of reading difficulties.

29. d.   Alzheimer's patients cannot recognize familiar persons (visual
          spatial disturbance), have impaired driving, misplace objects
          (spatial agnosia), do not recognize familiar objects (visual
          agnosia), are unable to draw or copy (constructional apraxia),
          and become lost or disoriented (environmental disorientation).

30. a.   With age, the fat layer beneath the epidermis thins. This can
          produce pressure sores on the bridge of the nose. To alleviate
          this, a small frame with a distance between lenses near the
          interpupillary distances and high index plastic will reduce
          weight. Silicone nose pads will more evenly distribute the
          weight.

31. c.   In general, defects tend to be tritanopic with a reduction in
          discrimination in the blue and blue-green regions of the
          spectrum.

32. e.   Possible postreceptor mechanisms for age-related loss could be
          due to reduced receptor pooling (note that there is an age-related
          loss of photoreceptors) due to reduced convergence to bipolar
          cells, ganglion cell loss, decreased response amplitude of the
          neurons, decreased levels of retinal neurotransmitters, cortical cell
          loss with resultant reduction in cortical magnification factor, and
          decrease in levels of cortical neurotransmitters. All of these do
          occur as a function of age, but the variability between individuals
          is great. (See, for example, Chapter 32 of Benjamin WJ, Borish
          IM: *Borish's clinical refraction,* Philadelphia, 1998, Saunders, or
          Chapter 10 of Norton TT, Corliss DA, Bailey JE: *The
          psychophysical measurement of visual function,* Boston, 2002,
          Butterworth-Heinemann.)

33. e. Psychophysical tests rely on the patient's subjective response. Many elderly subjects do not say that they detect a target (say a Snellen letter) until they are very sure. Older subjects tend to adopt a very conservative criterion and are not risk takers and will not report that they see a letter (or target) unless their sensory evidence is strong. Younger observers tend to have a more relaxed criterion and are more likely to guess.

34. b. The elderly tend to have more difficulties with dark adaptation. The thresholds tend to be higher with increasing age throughout the entire time course of dark adaptation, as well as at the end of the dark adaptation period. In general, the thresholds are elevated by approximately 1 to 2 log units.

35. c. With foveally fixated targets, the spatial contrast sensitivity declines primarily in the intermediate and high spatial frequencies but not at the low spatial frequencies. This is thought to be due to primarily optical factors (miosis, absorption, and light scattering). However, the difference (the reduction) is greatly magnified if testing occurs at low illuminance. The decline in contrast sensitivity can be offset partially by increasing the luminance level used in testing.

CHAPTER 36

Anomalies Secondary to Acquired Neurologic Impairment

Edward S. Bennett, Vasudevan Lakshminarayanan

1. The chief ocular symptom of trigeminal nerve disease is:
   a. vertigo
   b. corneal anesthesia
   c. Meniere's disease
   d. facial nerve palsy

2. The chief ophthalmoscopic sign of increased intracranial pressure is:
   a. blurring of disc margin
   b. venous congestion
   c. peripapilledema
   d. a, b, and c

3. Ophthalmic findings in myasthenia gravis occur early because:
   a. of the high nerve-to-muscle ratio in extraocular muscle
   b. of the low nerve-to-muscle ratio in extraocular muscle
   c. muscles are infiltrated with small round cells
   d. of the chronic and insidious onset

4. Supranuclear palsies are characterized by:
   a. diplopia
   b. visual field loss
   c. disturbances of eye movement systems
   d. Marcus Gunn pupil

5. Brainstem lesions result in:
   a. absence of suppression
   b. anomalous correspondence
   c. eccentric fixation
   d. a, b, and c

6. A bilateral visual field anomaly indicates the location of the problem as being:
    a. prechiasmal
    b. postchiasmal
    c. in the anterior radiations
    d. in the ganglion cell layer of the retina

7. An afferent papillary defect can be detected by studying the results from:
    a. a visual field examination
    b. swinging flashlight test
    c. vergence eye movements/phoria tests
    d. a, b, and c

8. Which one of the following is NOT a possible cause of an acquired neurologic palsy resulting in strabismus?
    a. Duane retraction syndrome
    b. trauma to the oculomotor nuclei
    c. brainstem tumor
    d. multiple sclerosis

9. Which one of the following is FALSE as it pertains to an acquired neurogenic palsy?
    a. noncomitant strabismus is likely
    b. amblyopia would be a common finding
    c. trauma is a common cause
    d. recent onset of diplopia is a common symptom

10. When questioning a patient who may have an acquired neurogenic ocular palsy, you should ask if the patient has a history of:
    a. head tilt
    b. headaches
    c. head trauma
    d. double vision
    e. a, b, c, and d

Answers

1. b. Corneal anesthesia is the chief ocular symptom of trigeminal nerve disease. The patient may also experience loss of facial and intraoral sensation and weakness of jaw closure. Local corneal anesthesia also occurs with the herpes simplex infection and following a variety of intraocular surgical procedures.

2. d. Papilledema is the chief ophthalmoscopic sign. The features could include all of the choices given as well as a loss of previously noted venous pulse, hyperemia, and peripapillary edema with concentric traction lines.

3. a. The mechanism seems to be an increase in circulating antibodies to acetylcholine receptors on an autoimmune basis. Bilateral ptosis or other extraocular muscle weakness occurs in about 90% of cases.

4. c. Supranuclear palsies are characterized by disturbances of the oculomotor systems: saccadic, vergence, pursuit, or vestibular movements.

5. d. Brainstem lesions often affect facial, auditory, vestibular, or trigeminal nerves; the pupil; and the medial longitudinal fasciculus.

6. b. A bilateral anomaly indicated that the problem occurs in the chiasma or beyond. Lesions of the optic tract and anterior radiations tend to be incongruous, and posterior lesions are congruous.

7. b. If there is a difference in the number of optic nerve axons carrying impulses from each retina, then light shined into the eye with fewer axons will cause a lesser amount of papillary constriction than will light shined into the other eye. This is the Marcus Gunn pupil.

8. a. Trauma to the oculomotor nuclei, a brainstem tumor, and multiple sclerosis, as well as neuronal tumors, vascular disorders, and myasthenia gravis, are all possible causes of acquired neurologic palsy. Duane retraction syndrome, characterized by the paradoxical co-contraction of the ipsilateral medial and lateral rectus muscles, is a congenital sixth nerve palsy.

9. b. Amblyopia is quite common in a developmental comitant strabismus but is rare in an acquired noncomitant strabismus. In the case of an acquired neurogenic palsy, trauma and neurologic systemic disease are common. In addition, recent onset of diplopia and an abnormal head tilt are common findings.

10.   e. As all of these findings may be present or certainly can be indicative of an acquired neurogenic ocular palsy; it is important to ask all of these questions in performing a comprehensive history on these patients.

CHAPTER 37

Inherited and Acquired Color Vision Disorders

Vasudevan Lakshminarayanan

1. According to Kollner's rule, inner retinal and optic nerve diseases result in:
   a. blue-yellow–type color vision defects
   b. red-green type–color vision defects
   c. achromatopsia
   d. a nonselective loss of color vision

2. In rod monochromacy, which of the following is FALSE?
   a. M and L cones are completely absent
   b. poor color discrimination is exhibited
   c. nystagmus is present
   d. condition is autosomal recessive

3. Xanthopsia:
   a. is a distortion of color vision
   b. is a form of chromatopsia
   c. can occur secondary to the administration of digitalis
   d. can occur in patients after fluorescein angiography

4. Colors that cannot be distinguished by dichromats lie along straight lines on the CIE color space and are called:
   a. confusion lines
   b. convergence lines
   c. copunctal lines
   d. neutral lines

5. Genetics research has shown that various congenital color vision defects can be attributed to:
   a. missing cone types
   b. missing or hybridization of the two X-linked cone photopigment genes
   c. variations in ocular media absorption spectra
   d. malfunctioning color opponent pathway

6. Anomalous trichromats can have:
   a. abnormal M-cone photopigment
   b. abnormal L-cone photopigment
   c. abnormal S-cone photopigment
   d. a and b
   e. b and c

7. On a Farnsworth Munsell FM-100 test, if the illumination level is reduced below the recommended level:
   a. there is an increase in the number of errors
   b. a tritan axis is revealed
   c. a deutan axis is revealed
   d. a protan axis is revealed

8. If on a FM-100 test the cap ordering is 7-9-8, the error score for the position 9 will be:
   a. 10
   b. 8
   c. 6
   d. 3

9. When producing a color match, the two colors that are perceptually identical but have different spectral compositions:
   a. are called isomers
   b. are called metamers
   c. satisfy the principle of univariance
   d. are not seen by anomalous dichromats

10. Which of the following is FALSE regarding congenital X-linked inherited color vision disorders?
    a. they are symmetric or equal in both eyes
    b. they are often blue-yellow–type defects
    c. they are stable throughout life
    d. they are almost always red-green–type defects

Answers

1. b. According to Kollner's rule, outer retinal and media changes result in blue-yellow color vision defects, whereas diseases of the inner retina, optic nerve, visual pathways, and visual cortex result in red-green defects. However, there are some important exceptions. (See Schneck M, Haegerstrom-Portnoy G: *Investig Ophthalmol Visual Sci* 38:2278-2289, 1997, Table 6-4; page 146 of Schwartz SH: *Visual perception,* ed 3, New York, 2004, McGraw-Hill; and page 280 of Norton TT, Corliss DA, Bailey JE: *The psychophysical measurement of visual function,* Boston, 2002, Butterworth Heinemann.)

2. a. This is the most common achromatopsia. Rod monochromats may have M and L cone types, but the numbers will be reduced. (See page 455 of Kaiser PK, Boynton RM: *Human color vision,* ed 2, 1996, Optical Society of America.)

3. e. Xanthopsia means yellow vision and is a form of chromatopsia, which are not true color vision defects. They do not typically produce a decreased ability to discriminate colors. (See, for example, page 146 of Schwartz SH: *Visual perception,* ed 3, New York, 2004, McGraw-Hill.)

4. a. Color confusion lines can be plotted on a CIE diagram. All colors falling on a confusion line are indistinguishable to a dichromat. The color confusion lines for deuteranopia, protanopia, and tritanopia all originate from a different copunctal point. (See, for example, Figure 8.21, page 272 of Norton TT, Corliss DA, Bailey JE: *The psychophysical measurement of visual function,* Boston, 2002, Butterworth Heinemann.)

5. b. It is found that that the highly homologous genes for M and L cone photopigment are positioned on the X chromosome in a head-to-tail tandem array. Erroneous crossover of genetic information could occur when the pair of X chromosomes align and exchange genetic information during meiosis. There could be intergenetic crossover, or there could be hybrid genes (fusion or chimeric genes) due to intragenetic crossover. (See discussion on pages 463-481 of Kaiser PK, Boynton RM: *Human color vision,* ed 2, 1996, Optical Society of America.)

6. d. Anomalous trichromats who have an abnormal M photopigment are deuteranomalous, whereas those with abnormal L photopigment are called protonamalous. (See Table 10.2, page 444, of Kaiser PK, Boynton RM: *Human color vision,* ed 2, 1996, Optical Society of America.)

7. a. As with all pseudoisochromatic plates, the FM-100 must be used with the appropriate illuminant and at the recommended illumination level.

8. d. The error score for each cap is the sum of the absolute differences between the number of that cap and the numbers of the adjacent caps. Here this is equal to $(9 - 7 = 2) + (9 - 8 = 1) = 3$.

9. b. Metamers by definition are two stimuli (or lights) that appear identical but are physically different (i.e., different spectral composition). (See, for example, page 228 in Norton TT, Corliss DA, Bailey JE: *The psychophysical measurement of visual function,* Boston, 2002, Butterworth Heinemann.)

10. b. Blue-yellow–type defects are usually acquired color defects. (See Table 8-6, page 276, Norton TT, Corliss DA, Bailey JE: *The psychophysical measurement of visual function,* Boston, 2002, Butterworth Heinemann.)

Part 4 Recommended Reading

Ball K, Beard B, Roenker D: Age and visual search: expanding the useful field of view. *J Am Optom Soc* 5:2210-2219, 1988.

Ball K, Owsley C: The useful field of view test: a new technique for evaluating age related declines in visual function. *J Am Optom Assoc* 64:71-79, 1993.

Benjamin WJ, Borish IM: *Borish's clinical refraction*, Philadelphia, 1998, Saunders.

Caird R, Pirie M, Ramsell TG: *Diabetes and the eye*, Oxford, 1969, Blackwell.

Enoch JM, Werner JG, Hagerstrom-Portnoy G et al: Forever young: visual functions not affected or minimally affected by aging. *J Gerontol Biol Sci* 54A:B336-B352, 1999.

Griffin JR, Grisham JD: *Binocular anomalies: diagnosis and vision therapy*, ed 4, Boston, 2002, Butterworth-Heinemann.

Kaiser PK, Boynton RM: *Human color vision,* ed 2, 1996, Optical Society of America.

Liu GT, Volpe NJ, Galetta SL: *Neuro-ophthalmology diagnosis and management,* Philadelphia, 2001, Saunders.

Millodot M: Influence of age on the sensitivity of the cornea. *Invest Ophthalmol Vis Sci* 16:240-272, 1977.

Norton TT, Corliss DA, Bailey JE: *The psychophysical measurement of visual function,* Boston, 2002, Butterworth Heinemann.

Rosenbloom AA, Morgan MW: *Vision and aging,* ed 2, Boston, 1993, Butterworth Heinemann.

Schwartz SH: *Visual perception,* ed 3, New York, 2004, McGraw-Hill.

Schwartz B, Kern J: Age, increased ocular and blood pressures and retinal and disc fluorescein angiogram. *Arch Ophthalmol* 98:1980-1986, 1980.

Weale RA: *The senescence of human vision,* New York, 1992, Oxford University Press.

Weleber RA: The effect of age in human cone and rod Ganzfeld electroretinograms. *Invest Ophthalmol* 20:392-399, 1981.

Public Health

Epidemiology

Chris Woodruff

1. The proportion of a population with a particular disease or condition at a particular point in time is known as:
    a. incidence
    b. prevalence
    c. relative risk
    d. odds ratio

2. A prospective study of lung cancer and cigarette smoking revealed that 200 of 500 smokers developed lung cancer while only 25 of 500 nonsmokers developed the disease. According to this study, the relative risk attributed to cigarette smoking is:
    a. 0.40
    b. 2
    c. 4
    d. 8

3. The probability that a healthy person will develop a disease or condition during a specific time period can be quantified using:
    a. incidence rate
    b. odds ratio
    c. prevalence
    d. relative risk

4. The ability of a screening test to predict those individuals with the disease or condition in question is called:
    a. sensitivity
    b. specificity
    c. predictive value
    d. yield

5. The yield of a screening test is affected by all of the following EXCEPT:
   a. sensitivity of the test
   b. specificity of the test
   c. prevalence of unrecognized disease
   d. frequency of screening

6. The probability that an individual with a positive finding on a screening test actually has the disease in question is determined by:
   a. sensitivity
   b. specificity
   c. predictive value
   d. odds ratio

7. The study of school-aged children that determined that modified clinical technique (MCT) is the best screening method for identifying vision disorders in this population was:
   a. Baltimore Eye Study
   b. Framingham Eye Study
   c. Orinda Study
   d. Beaver Dam Eye Study

8. Which of the following studies was designed to determine the prevalence of eye diseases in an adult population?
   a. Baltimore Eye Study
   b. Beaver Dam Eye Study
   c. Framingham Eye Study
   d. Orinda Study

9. An advantage of prospective study design compared with retrospective study design is:
   a. generally shorter duration
   b. less expensive
   c. fewer problems with subject retention
   d. information given on incidence rates

10. The leading cause of mortality in the United States (for all ages) is:
    a. cerebrovascular disease
    b. infectious disease
    c. malignant neoplastic disease
    d. heart disease

Answers

1. b. Prevalence is the number of existing cases of a disease or condition divided by the population of interest. Incidence is the number of new cases of a disease or condition for a particular time period.

2. d. Relative risk is found by dividing the incidence rate of those exposed by the incidence rate of those not exposed. The incidence rate for the exposed is 200/500. The incidence rate of those not exposed is 25/500.

3. a. The incidence rate is determined by dividing the number of new cases during a specific time period (usually 1 year) by the population at risk. Incidence provides a way to quantify the risk of developing disease during a specific time period.

4. a. Sensitivity is determined by dividing the number of true-positive test results by the number of individuals who actually have the disease (true-positives and false-negatives). Sensitivity is a measure of how good the test is at correctly identifying those with disease. Specificity is a measure of how good the test is at correctly identifying those individuals without the disease.

5. b. Yield is defined as the number of new cases brought to treatment as a result of the screening test. Sensitivity will determine the number of persons referred for additional testing. Specificity is a measurement of how well the screening test can predict those who do not have the disease or condition in question and therefore does not affect the yield of the screening test. Yield will be affected by the portion of the population with the disease or condition (prevalence) and how often the screening is performed.

6. c. The predictive value (of a positive test) tells us how likely a person who has a positive test finding is of having the disease or condition and is determined by dividing the number of true positives by the total number of positive test results (true-positives and false-positives).

7. c. The Orinda Study evaluated a number of vision screening batteries in terms of effectiveness and efficiency on a group of school-aged children. Although the MCT was not the least expensive method and required an eye care professional for administration, it was determined to be the best method available for screening school-aged children for vision disorders.

8.   c.   The purpose of the Framingham Eye Study was to look at the prevalence of eye disease among the survivors of the Framingham Heart Study. The Orinda Study was concerned with vision screening and vision disorders in school-aged children. The Baltimore and Beaver Dam studies were concerned with blindness and visual impairment in adults.

9.   d.   Prospective studies are generally longer in duration and more expensive than retrospective studies. There is also the problem of retaining subjects for the duration of the study. One of the advantages of prospective design over retrospective design is the ability to determine incidence rates.

10.   d.   The three leading causes of death (for all age groups combined) in order are (1) heart disease, (2) cancer, and (3) stroke.

CHAPTER 39

Biostatistics and Measurement

Chris Woodruff

1. The best measure of central tendency in a dataset with a large standard deviation is:
    a. median
    b. mode
    c. mean
    d. variance

2. Choosing controls for a case-control study of VDT use and vision problems from participants in a community health screening may create:
    a. recall bias
    b. selection bias
    c. information bias
    d. interviewer bias

3. Which of the following is TRUE regarding validity and reliability?
    a. validity refers to accuracy; reliability to repeatability
    b. validity refers to repeatability; reliability to accuracy
    c. validity and reliability are both measures of accuracy
    d. validity and reliability are both measures of repeatability

4. If the mean intraocular pressure (IOP) in a normally distributed population of individuals without glaucoma is 14 mm Hg and the standard deviation is 2 mm Hg, what percentage of the population will have an IOP greater than 18 mm Hg?
    a. 0.5%
    b. 1.0%
    c. 2.5%
    d. 5.0%

5. A study comparing the efficacy of two glaucoma medications has a
    statistical power of 0.80. The chance of failing to detect a difference in
    efficacy when a difference does indeed exist is:
    a. 2%
    b. 8%
    c. 20%
    d. 80%

Answers

1. a. In a dataset with outliers (extreme values), and consequently a higher standard deviation, the median provides a better measure of central tendency than the mean or the mode.

2. b. Selection bias occurs because of flaws in the participant selection process. Controls should be selected randomly from the population and have the same exposure level as the population. Individuals attending a health fair may not be representative of the population.

3. a. Validity is a measurement of accuracy and is concerned with how close the results are compared to the actual value. Reliability is a measure of repeatability and is concerned with obtaining the same results each time a test or procedure is performed.

4. c. In a normally distributed population, approximately 95% of the population will be within 2 standard deviations of the mean. Of the 5% more than 2 standard deviations from the mean, half (2.5%) will be more than 2 standard deviations above the mean and half will be more than 2 standard deviations below the mean. Because 18 mm Hg is 2 standard deviations above the mean, 2.5% of this population will have an IOP greater than 18 mm Hg.

5. c. A Type II error is failing to detect a difference when one exists. Statistical power is $1 - -\beta$. Because β is the risk of committing a Type II error and the statistical power is 0.80, β must be 0.20, or 20%.

Environmental Vision

Chris Woodruff

1. Which requires impact resistance for street eyewear?
   a. American National Standards Institute (ANSI)
   b. Occupational Safety and Health Administration (OSHA)
   c. Food and Drug Administration (FDA)
   d. Federal Trade Commission (FTC)

2. The majority of work-related eye injuries are caused by:
   a. flying or falling objects
   b. chemicals
   c. ultraviolet radiation
   d. heat

3. In normal indoor lighting, we are exposed to approximately:
   a. 5 to 200 foot candles
   b. 100 to 1,000 foot candles
   c. 500 to 5,000 foot candles
   d. 5,000 to 10,000 foot candles

4. Optimal reading performance is achieved with letter size:
   a. at the visual acuity level
   b. one line above the visual acuity level
   c. two to three times the visual acuity level
   d. five times the visual acuity level

5. Which of the following will NOT help reduce the symptoms of a patient who *complains* of eyestrain when using a computer with a CRT display?
   a. elevate the monitor so that it is 10 to 15 degrees above the line of sight
   b. prescribe correcting lenses for −0.50D of uncorrected astigmatism
   c. prescribe an antireflective coating for their spectacle lenses
   d. treat the patient's convergence insufficiency with vision therapy

1. c. The FDA requires that street eyewear be impact resistant. ANSI provides standards for dress and safety eyewear. OSHA is concerned with the health and safety of the workplace. The FTC is concerned with fair trade and consumer protection.

2. a. Almost 70% of work-related injuries are caused by flying or falling objects or sparks. Chemical contact is responsible for one in five work-related eye injuries.

3. a. During the daylight hours, the illumination of the earth's surface is generally between 500 and 10,000 foot candles; however, indoor light levels are generally 5 to 200 foot candles.

4. c. Studies show that optimal reading performance occurs when the reading material is sized two and a half to three times the visual acuity level. Letter sizes smaller or greater than this can have a negative impact on reading performance.

5. a. For maximum comfort, the computer screen should be located 10 to 20 degrees below the line of sight. Even low amounts of uncorrected refractive error can produce symptoms with computer use. An antireflective coating can improve image resolution. Accommodative and convergence problems can create symptoms of eyestrain and therefore should be properly treated.

CHAPTER 41

Health Care Policy and Administration

Chris Woodruff

1. The practice setting for the majority of optometrists in the United States is:
   a. private practice
   b. employed by ophthalmologists
   c. HMO
   d. retail practice

2. The agency responsible for the licensing of optometrists in the United States is:
   a. Department of Health and Human Services
   b. the American Optometric Association
   c. the states' boards of optometry
   d. Federal Trade Commission (FTC)

3. The health care payment mechanism in which the provider is contracted to provide services on a prepaid basis for a specific time period is called:
   a. an indemnity plan
   b. a preferred provider plan
   c. a capitation plan
   d. a service plan

4. The U.S. Public Health Service has determined that a ratio of one optometrist per 15,000 is adequate to meet the needs of a given population. If the utilization rate for all age groups in the population is 0.20, each optometrist must be able to provide:
   a. 1,500 encounters per year
   b. 2,000 encounters per year
   c. 3,000 encounters per year
   d. 7,500 encounters per year

5. Using noncontact tonometry at a health fair to screen for glaucoma is a form of:
   a. primary prevention
   b. primary care
   c. secondary prevention
   d. secondary care

6. Which BEST describes the current trend in reducing the impact of untreated vision disorders among school-aged children?
   a. government-mandated periodic eye examination
   b. increased funding for school-based vision screening
   c. greater utilization of eye care professionals in school screening
   d. increased reimbursements for those providing Medicaid vision services

7. In 2001, the name of the federal agency responsible for administering the Medicare program in the United States was changed to the Centers for Medicare and Medicaid Services. This agency was formerly known as:
   a. the Government Accounting Office (GAO)
   b. the Office of the Inspector General (OIG)
   c. the Health Care Financing Administration (HCFA)
   d. the Office of Health and Human Services (HHS)

8. The managed care system in which patients choose from a panel of participating doctors and receive reduced fees or a greater package of benefits if they use a panel doctor is known as:
   a. health maintenance organization (HMO)
   b. preferred provider organization (PPO)
   c. independent practitioner association (IPA)
   d. indemnity plan (IP)

9. Which statement is most accurate concerning health care spending in the United States?
   a. health care costs are rising slower than the rate of inflation
   b. health care costs are rising at about the rate of inflation
   c. health care costs are rising faster than the rate of inflation
   d. health care costs should not be compared with inflation

10. Enforcement of compliance with the Health Insurance Portability and Accountability Act (HIPAA) is the responsibility of:
    a. The Federal Trade Commission (FTC)
    b. The Food & Drug Administration (FDA)
    c. Health and Human Services (HHS)
    d. Centers for Disease Control and Prevention (CDC)

Answers

1. a. The majority of optometrists are engaged in private practice. A small number of optometrists work for HMOs and ophthalmologists. The percentage of optometrists in retail practice has increased over the past several decades.

2. c. The federal government provides police powers to the states. Through these powers, the practice of optometry is regulated. The licensure of optometrists is controlled by each state's board of optometry.

3. c. Capitation is a payment mechanism in which the provider is paid in advance to provide care for a specific time period.

4. c. To determine the number of patient encounters each optometrist must be able to handle, multiply the number of potential patients (15,000) by the utilization rate. The utilization rate tells us the percentage of the population that is expected to require care during the year.

5. c. Screening is not the same as providing health care but instead is a form of prevention. Primary prevention involves specific protective measures against the development of disease. Secondary prevention involves the early detection and prompt treatment of disease.

6. a. There is a trend toward requiring eye examinations for preschool children. This will reduce the need for school vision screenings.

7. c. The Health Care Financing Administration became the Centers for Medicare and Medicaid Services on July 1, 2001. The emphasis is now on improving the quality of care beneficiaries receive.

8. b. In a preferred provider organization, the patient is given greater freedom of choice in selecting a provider. If the patient chooses a preferred provider, they will receive reduced fees or a more generous package of benefits.

9. c. Health care costs are increasing at a rate that exceeds the rate of inflation. Health care spending is now greater than 14% of gross domestic product (GDP). The cost of health care is increasing 7% to 8% per year.

10.   c.   Health and Human Services is the agency responsible for HIPAA compliance. The FTC enforces a variety of federal antitrust and consumer protection laws. The FDA is responsible for protecting the public health by ensuring the safety of drugs, medical devices, food, and cosmetics. The CDC is the federal agency charged with protecting the health and safety of the American public.

Part 5 Recommended Reading

Johnson GJ, Weale R, Minassian, DC, West SK: *The epidemiology of eye disease,* ed 2, London, 2003, Arnold Publishers.

Newcomb RD, Marshall EC: *Public health and community optometry,* ed 2, Boston, 1990, Butterworth-Heinemann.

Pitts DG, Kleinstein RN: *Environmental vision,* Boston, 1993, Butterworth-Heinemann.

Legal and Ethical Issues

CHAPTER 42

Licensure and Governmental Regulation of Optometry

John G. Classé

1. The legal authority for the licensure of optometrists may be found in which of the following sources of law?
   a. state statutes
   b. federal laws
   c. state boards of optometry
   d. federal administrative agencies

2. The powers granted to state boards of optometry do NOT include:
   a. the duty to investigate violations of the optometry law
   b. the authority to enact laws
   c. the right to initiate litigation (file lawsuits)
   d. the right to hold disciplinary hearings

3. The regulation of impact standards for protective eyewear in the workplace ("safety glasses") is the responsibility of the:
   a. U.S. Food and Drug Administration
   b. Occupational Safety and Health Administration
   c. Federal Trade Commission
   d. Drug Enforcement Administration

4. The Americans With Disabilities Act does NOT regulate which of the following?
   a. applications for employment by individuals with disabilities
   b. the determination of reasonable "accommodations" for workers with disabilities
   c. assessment of impairment for persons with disabilities
   d. the dismissal of employees with disabilities

5. Which of the following tests is NOT used when assessing permanent vision impairment according to the guidelines of the American Medical Association's *Guides to the Evaluation of Permanent Impairment*?
    a. determination of best corrected visual acuity
    b. measurement of the field of vision
    c. plotting of diplopia in nine positions of gaze
    d. calculating the impairment of the whole person

Answers

1. a. Because the U.S. Constitution contains no provisions for the regulation of health care, licensure and discipline of optometrists and other health care providers are performed at the state level, through laws passed by state legislatures. State boards of optometry administer laws but are not the source of licensure. Federal agencies provide regulation but do not affect licensure.

2. b. Boards of optometry are given authority to pass rules or regulations that facilitate the administration of laws duly enacted by the legislature. Thus, the law-making authority is invested in the legislature, but boards can investigate violations, hold disciplinary hearings, and file lawsuits. But they cannot "make" law.

3. b. Under federal law, the impact standards for industrial strength ("safety") lenses and the workplace requirements for the wear of "safety glasses" are the responsibility of the Occupational Safety and Health Administration.

4. c. The Americans With Disabilities Act was passed to eliminate discrimination against disabled individuals in applications for employment and in the performance of their jobs. An employee with a disability must be provided a reasonable "accommodation" if doing so would permit that worker to perform vital job functions. If a disabled employee cannot perform the vital tasks necessary, even with an "accommodation," the law provides for dismissal. However, the ADA does not provide for the assessment of an applicant's or worker's disability by the employer.

5. c. The AMA's *Guides to the Evaluation of Permanent Impairment* describes the methods to be used for determining the level of impairment that a person has sustained. The guidelines for vision impairment were significantly amended in the fifth edition, to include just two principal measures: visual acuity and visual field. Binocularity (diplopia) is no longer a principal measure, just an "individual adjustment," and so plotting of diplopia (necessary under previous *Guides*) is no longer a requirement. Calculation of the impairment of the "whole person" remains the end result of the evaluation process.

CHAPTER 43

Standards of Professional Ethics

John G. Classé

1. "Ethics" is considered to be:
    a. based on legal principles of "right" and "wrong"
    b. the fundamental basis for the conduct of a trade
    c. a moral concept
    d. less demanding in terms of conduct than "law"

2. The guiding principle of ethics for health care providers is to:
    a. do no wrong
    b. serve the interests of patients before one's own
    c. avoid derogatory comments about other professionals
    d. observe the tenets of *caveat emptor* ("let the buyer beware")

3. Which of the following has historically been a distinguishing characteristic of professionalism for health care providers?
    a. freedom to practice in the environment of the provider's choosing
    b. duty to respect the confidentiality of patient information
    c. right to exercise freedom of speech in promoting oneself as a provider
    d. obligation to provide services based on the patient's ability to pay

4. Advertising has long been held to be incompatible with professionalism. Which of the following is NOT a reason that has been used to criticize the use of advertising by professionals?
    a. it is too easily made misleading to a lay public
    b. it is at odds with the premise that a professional's reputation for competence should be the reason to seek the professional's services
    c. it is not a cost-effective use of monetary resources
    d. it is used to emphasize cheapness rather than quality

5. Oaths (such as the Optometric Oath) have been used by medicine and the health care professions primarily to serve which of the following purposes?
    a. set ideals of conduct for professionals to aspire to follow
    b. establish enforceable practice guidelines
    c. reduce competition by creating rules by which all professionals have to abide
    d. promote the professions to the public

Answers

1. c. Ethics is a moral concept and provides rules of conduct for professionals (not tradesmen); hence, it is not legal in nature and in fact almost always requires a higher level of conduct than is required by the law.

2. b. Ethics requires that a health care professional put the interests of patients before the professional's own. This means always making decisions based on the benefit to patients rather than the benefit to the practitioner. Although "first do no wrong" is a time-tested phrase from the Hippocratic Oath, it is not the key underlying concept of professional ethics. *Caveat emptor* is the philosophy of the marketplace, not of professionalism. Although it is considered ethical to avoid making derogatory comments, especially about one's colleagues, doing so is not the foundation of ethical conduct.

3. b. Historically, the duty to respect confidentiality goes back more than 2,000 years, while choice of work environment and use of advertising are ideas about a tenth that old. The setting of fees is an ethical issue of long standing, but one precept of that issue has been that services should be rendered without regard to a patient's ability to pay. Providing services (or not doing so) based on a patient's ability to pay is the opposite of that.

4. c. Advertising has been deemed incompatible with professionalism because it typically emphasizes cost (cheapness) or personal promotion (which can be misleading). The traditional means of building a practice has been by word of mouth, which is based on an individual's personal experience with a practitioner and not due to the pronouncements of an advertisement. The one criticism against advertising that has not been used is cost—it is understood that cost is an element of an advertising campaign.

5. a. The Hippocratic Oath describes the type of conduct that a physician is expected to display when attending to patients. It was an attempt to set ideals for physicians to emulate, not to stifle competition, for it could not be enforced by punishment of physicians who did not heed it. The Optometric Oath is similar in purpose, and although it admittedly "promotes" the profession to the public, its principal purpose is to set ideals for practitioners.

Doctor-Patient Relationship

John G. Classé

1. Which of the following disclosures, if made by a doctor without the consent of the patient, would constitute a breach of confidentiality?
   a. reporting a finding of communicable disease in a patient to the spouse
   b. submitting information as required by law that a patient no longer meets the vision qualifications to operate a motor vehicle
   c. replying to an insurance company's request for examination information about a patient who is a policyholder
   d. providing examination findings about a child to the child's parent

2. If there is a legal proceeding involving a doctor's patient, because of the "doctor-patient privilege," testimony by the doctor concerning the care rendered to the patient:
   a. must be provided at the proceeding
   b. is allowed if the patient agrees to let the doctor testify
   c. can be divulged if the doctor believes the information is not confidential
   d. cannot be divulged because a doctor cannot be compelled to disclose patient information even in a legal proceeding

3. Defamation is a legal action in which damages are sought for:
   a. public disclosure of private information
   b. negligence
   c. disclosure of confidential information without consent
   d. injury to reputation

4. Which of the following acts, committed by a doctor in private practice, would constitute invasion of privacy?
   a. displaying in the doctor's office a photograph autographed by a celebrity patient
   b. publishing a newspaper story with quotations provided by a patient
   c. including a picture of a patient's face in a journal article written by the doctor
   d. using a patient's refractive data in a research paper compiled by the doctor

5. The records compiled by an optometrist in private practice are the property of:
   a. the optometrist
   b. the patient
   c. the optometrist and patient jointly
   d. none of the above

6. For legal purposes, the preferable way to correct an error in a patient record is to:
   a. redo the record so that it is correct
   b. make no changes or corrections on the record itself but rather use a separate page
   c. draw a line through the incorrect data, initial and date it, and write in the correct information
   d. eradicate the incorrect data, enter the correct information, and note the date the change was made

7. Which of the following statements about the Federal Trade Commission's "eyeglasses" rule is NOT correct?
   a. the patient is entitled to a copy of the spectacle prescription if there is a change in sphere power, cylinder power or axis, or add power
   b. the spectacle prescription can contain an expiration date
   c. reasonable limitations (e.g., "polycarbonate plastic only") can be included on the spectacle prescription
   d. the doctor can charge a fee for verifying spectacles obtained from a third-party dispenser on the doctor's prescription

8. The specific (minimum) information that must be included in a spectacle prescription is determined by:
   a. the FTC "eyeglasses" rules only
   b. the provisions of state law only
   c. both the FTC "eyeglasses" rules and the provisions of state law, if applicable

9. Under the requirements of HIPAA, an optometrist needs a signed "authorization" form from the patient to release information to third parties about:
   a. health care operations (i.e., for referral to another practitioner)
   b. results of past examinations
   c. treatment provided to the patient
   d. payment for services

10. Which of the following statements about HIPAA is NOT correct?
    a. doctors must amend records if patients ask for them to be changed based upon perceived errors
    b. all practices must have a "privacy officer"
    c. patients have the right to inspect and copy their records
    d. doctors can have patients waive their HIPAA rights under some circumstances

Answers

1. c. Breach of confidentiality occurs when truthful confidential information (such as examination findings) is disclosed to a third party without consent. The law may require information to be disclosed (such as for a driver with reduced acuity) or may permit it in certain instances (communicable diseases, children's examination results), but if there is no legal basis for the disclosure, it is improper. Thus, insurance companies or other third parties do not have a legal right to confidential information unless the person involved consents to the disclosure.

2. b. The "doctor-patient privilege" is a statutory provision found in most states that pertains to the disclosure by doctors in legal proceedings of the information obtained during the examination of a patient. The privilege can only be exerted by the patient (not the doctor), and if the patient asserts it, the doctor is barred from testifying or otherwise providing the information. Very few states allow the privilege to be used if the doctor involved is an optometrist.

3. d. Defamation occurs when Person A communicates information about Person B (the "publication") to Person C (or to many persons) and as a consequence of this publication there is resultant injury to the reputation of Person B. The communication does not have to be negligently published to be actionable. Disclosure of confidential information without consent is a different offense, known as breach of the duty to respect confidentiality. Public disclosure of private facts is an invasion of privacy.

4. c. There are four types of conduct, if committed by a doctor, that would constitute invasion of privacy: use of a patient's name or likeness without consent, release of publicity that places a patient in a false light, public disclosure of private facts about a patient, and intrusion on a patient's privacy by a third party. The first type, use of name or likeness without consent, cannot occur if the patient has willingly signed a photograph or provided quotations for an article. Nor can it occur where information is used—such as refractive data—that does not identify the patient. If a facial photograph is published without consent, however, even in a professional journal, it may be held that such publication constitutes an invasion of privacy.

5. a. A private practitioner owns the patient records compiled by that practitioner while providing care to patients. Patients have a right of access to the information, however, even though they have no ownership right. HIPAA has greatly reinforced this right of access to information in the record but has not altered ownership provisions.

6. c. The best way to correct an entry in a record is to draw a line through the incorrect entry, initial and date it, write in the correct information, and if necessary add an explanation as to why the correction is being made.

7. a. The FTC's "eyeglasses" rule obligates optometrists to give patients a copy of the spectacle prescription whether or not there is a change in it. No differences in power or axis are required. The prescription must contain an expiration date, and reasonable limitations (such as a specific lens material) are permissible. An optometrist can charge a fee for verifying spectacles based on the optometrist's prescription but obtained from a different dispenser.

8. c. The exact information (e.g., lens powers, expiration date, signature) that must be included in a spectacle prescription is not described in the FTC's "eyeglasses" rule. Rather, the rule contains a statement that the information provided must be sufficient for the patient to obtain spectacles if the prescription is presented to a dispenser. The FTC rule also says that if state law specifies the minimum information to be included in a spectacle prescription, then that information has to be provided. Thus, both federal and state laws may determine the information to be included in a spectacle prescription.

9. b. HIPAA requires practitioners using electronic submissions to impose a privacy policy that safeguards the confidentiality of identifiable personal health care information. Patients must be informed of the policy (and may read it if they desire) and must sign a form indicating that they understand it. Practitioners are then permitted to use examination information without further consent for billing and payment, treatment, and "health care operations," a term that includes referrals to other practitioners. Examination data can be shared with the other practitioner without asking the patient for permission. If there is a request for information that is not related to billing and payment, treatment, or health care operations, such as a request for past examination results from a third party, the patient must be informed of the request and asked to sign an "authorization" that permits the information's release for this specific purpose.

10.   d.   HIPAA requires doctors' offices to have a "privacy officer" who is
expected to implement the HIPAA rules and train employees so
they understand them. The act allows patients access to their
records, including the right to copy them, and permits patients to
ask doctors to change the records if they believe the records are
incorrect. However, the act states that patients cannot be required
to waive their HIPAA rights as a condition for examination by the
doctor.

Professional Liability

John G. Classé

1. To create the doctor-patient relationship:
   a. a fee for services must be charged
   b. there must be some direct communication between the two persons involved
   c. the doctor must have examined the patient
   d. the persons involved must have intended to be doctor and patient

2. Proof of negligence does NOT ordinarily include evidence to establish:
   a. damages
   b. a breach of the standard of care
   c. proximate cause, which links the conduct of the defendant doctor to the injury suffered by the patient
   d. an intent to commit the act that resulted in injury

3. To satisfy federal impact-resistance standards, dress ophthalmic lenses must be no less than a minimum of:
   a. 2.0 mm
   b. 2.5 mm
   c. 3.0 mm
   d. there is no minimum lens thickness requirement for dress lenses

4. Under premises liability law, an optometrist in an office building would NOT be responsible for an injury to a patient occurring:
   a. in areas of ingress and egress to the office
   b. from a defective piece of ophthalmic equipment used during the examination
   c. from a "slip and fall" in the reception room
   d. as the result of an obvious danger outside the office

5. Which of the following is NOT a requirement of the doctrine of informed consent?
   a. discussion of the risks of treatment
   b. discussion of alternatives to treatment
   c. discussion of the expected outcomes of treatment
   d. discussion of the anticipated costs of treatment

Answers

1. d. To create a doctor-patient relationship, the two parties must intend for there to be one. The test is objective: if an observer would reasonably have concluded from what was said and done that one party intended to be doctor and the other patient, then the relationship is formed. However, no fee is necessary (gratuitous services create the relationship), there does not need to be an examination (a telephone conversation will suffice), and in fact the doctor and patient do not even have to meet face-to-face (examples include radiologists and pathologists).

2. d. Proof of negligence requires that evidence be presented to establish: there was a doctor-patient relationship, the doctor deviated from the standard of care, there was physical injury to the patient, and there was a legal link ("proximate cause") between what the doctor did (or did not do) and the injury. Intent to commit the act that results in injury is not necessary. Negligence results from a failure to act as a reasonable person would have acted under the circumstances, thereby creating a risk of injury that results in damages.

3. d. The impact resistance standards for dress lenses are set by the U.S. Food and Drug Administration and reflected in ANSI standards Z80.1 (prescription) and Z80.3 (plano), which require that a drop ball test be administered. There is no minimum thickness requirement.

4. d. Under premises liability law, an optometrist in possession of land is under a duty to make the premises safe by conducting inspections and discovering patent (obvious) defects or latent (hidden) defects that a reasonable inspection would have revealed. This duty extends to entry and exit ways (areas of ingress and egress), the office premises (including furniture and equipment), and even outside areas such as a parking lot. If the danger is obvious, however, such as ice and snow on steps, and the visitor fails to take notice or exercise reasonable care, the optometrist will not be held liable for injury.

5. d. The doctrine of informed consent obligates a health care provider to: describe the risks of a proposed treatment; discuss the alternatives to that treatment; and review the expected outcomes of the treatment. It does not require a discussion of the costs involved in the treatment, although that is always a good idea.

Part 6 Recommended Reading

Classé JG: *Legal aspects of optometry,* Boston, 1989, Butterworth.

Classé JG, Thal LS, Kamen RD, Rounds RS, Association of Practice Management Educators: *Business aspects of optometry,* Philadelphia, 2004, Elsevier.

Index